Schizophrenia

A Practical Primer

Ravinder Reddy MD
Associate Professor
Department of Psychiatry
University of Pittsburgh
Western Psychiatric Institute & Clinic
Pittsburgh, PA, USA

Matcheri Keshavan MD
Associate Chair and Professor
Department of Psychiatry & Behavioral Neuroscience
Wayne State University
Detroit, MI, USA

Foreword by
Professor Robin M. Murray

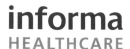

informa
HEALTHCARE

First published in the United Kingdom in 2006 by Informa Healthcare, an imprint of Informa UK Limited, 2–4 Park Square, Milton Park, Abingdon, Oxon OX14 4RN

Tel.:   +44 (0)20 7017 6000
Fax.:   +44 (0)20 7017 6699
E-mail: info.medicine@tandf.co.uk
Website: http://www.tandf.co.uk/medicine

A CIP record for this book is available from the British Library.
Library of Congress Cataloging-in-Publication Data

Data available on application

ISBN 10 1–841–84529–9
ISBN 13 978–1–841–84529–6

Distributed in North and South America by
Taylor & Francis
2000 NW Corporate Blvd
Boca Raton, FL 33431, USA

Within Continental USA
Tel: 800 272 7737; Fax: 800 374 3401
Outside Continental USA
Tel: 561 994 0555; Fax: 561 361 6018
E-mail: orders@crcpress.com

Distributed in the rest of the world by
Thomson Publishing Services
Cheriton House
North Way
Andover, Hampshire SP10 5BE, UK
Tel.: +44 (0)1264 332424
E-mail: salesorder.tandf@thomsonpublishingservices.co.uk

Composition by Wearset Ltd, Boldon, Tyne and Wear, UK
Printed and bound by MPG Books Ltd, Bodmin, Cornwall, UK

Dedication

We dedicate this book to the many patients and their relatives who helped us become better clinicians, to our students who helped us become better teachers, to our parents who helped us become better persons and to our wives and children for their unstinting support and encouragement.

Ravinder Reddy and Matcheri Keshavan

Contents

Appendices

Foreword

Schizophrenia can ruin the lives of those who develop it, and often dismays, and occasionally frightens, the friends and relatives of sufferers. It is one of the top ten causes of disability in developed countries, and affects as many as 50 million people worldwide. Thus, all kinds of health professionals, not just psychiatrists, need to be able to recognize schizophrenia, and to arrange treatment for it. Diagnosis is important as misdiagnosis can have serious consequences, yet it requires considerable skill to assess psychotic phenomena. Furthermore, as befits an illness at the interface between the brain and the social environment, treatment requires not just an understanding of psychopharmacology, but also of psychosocial interventions, and how they best work together to facilitate recovery.

The challenge, therefore, is how to teach the science and art of assessment and treatment of schizophrenia in a readily accessible manner. Drs Reddy and Keshavan have admirably accomplished this task. They are academics with many years of clinical experience, and have therefore been able to distill into this primer, the essence of the practical information that is required to work with patients with schizophrenia. The book is a deceptively easy read, but it is full of up-to-date information on all the topics that are required for the beginning mental health worker. In particular, the book is brought alive by the use of brief clinical vignettes ("clinical moments") along with questions for the reader. The authors have also packed the book with handy clinical notes and mnemonics, and the chapter on the history of schizophrenia is enlivened with drawings of the main historical figures!

Other aspects of this book further enhance its value. It utilizes a *phase of illness* approach to management, a better reflection of the reality of the disorder. There are also chapters on topics that are very important in practice, but are often neglected: communicating with families, role of culture, spirituality and religion, treatment nonadherence, and suboptimal treatment response. The authors have managed to pack into this modestly sized book the management of many drug side effects, a glossary of terms with over 150 definitions, and appendices that includes a listing of medications, further reading and websites.

In short, this book is authored by gifted clinicians and creative teachers who show a deep understanding of schizophrenia and respect for those who suffer from it. They have worked with patients in three continents and therefore bring a broad perspective to their advice. This practical primer will gently but clearly guide the beginning clinician from uncertainty to a sense of competence in working with patients and their families. I congratulate Ravinder Reddy and Matcheri Keshavan on their fine contribution to helping a future generation of mental health professionals.

Robin M. Murray
Professor of Psychiatry
Institute of Psychiatry
London, UK

Introduction

What this book is about

Everyone has heard of schizophrenia and many believe they understand it. However, lay notions are frequently at odds with what is known about schizophrenia by the clinicians and researchers who deal with this distressing disorder and, most importantly, by the patients and their families who are burdened by it.

In this *Primer* we aim to convey information about schizophrenia to those who are either required to work with patients having this disorder or are interested to do so. Before starting to write this book, we reflected on our many years of teaching about psychosis and schizophrenia to physicians, medical students, nurses, social workers, and other students. Invariably, we were reminded of the many questions asked by our students, patients, and their families; this provided both material and motivation to embark on this project. From this exercise emerged a set of principles about how we wished to transmit the information. We refer to this set of principles (our brief you might say) as BRIEFCase:

Brevity
Readability
Immediate utility
Essential material
Fun
Case-driven

Brevity
We aim at conveying information in few words, in order to save time, trees and toting, all of which need saving.

Readability

Too few words – telegraphic prose – can be tough to read. Thus, we aim at being readable, yet brief.

Immediate utility

Our intent is to arm you with information that mimics typical progression of clinical skills and knowledge base. For example, knowing that schizophrenia all over the world has similar presentation is important theoretically, but doesn't help in talking to the patient who is sitting across you. Thus, we did something novel – we moved the 'scientific' or *informational* chapters to the back of the book. The early chapters are *instructive*, the clinical stuff we think you need to know first.

Essential material

Determining what constitutes essential material was our greatest challenge. We are certain that we have missed material that others might consider essential. However, we do believe there to be enough substance in this book, in accord with the principles of BRIEFCase, to make you comfortable assessing and treating patients with schizophrenia. The intent of this book – a primer – is to provide enough information to help you on your way to the next level of clinical and scientific sophistication (and benefit from the many excellent advanced texts available on the subject).

Fun

We don't necessarily mean funny. We simply hope that reading this book will be enjoyable.

Case-driven

We are convinced that learning and teaching are best done at the bedside. The next best approach may be the use of appropriate case material presented in the form of a 'teachable moment'.

How to use this book (besides simply reading it)

Case scenarios

A brief (we mean brief) description of a clinical scenario is provided in a text box. Almost always a question accompanies the case – multiple choice or open ended. These questions are designed to sharpen your clinical thinking, not necessarily to help you pass exams. We suggest that you read the case, answer the question, and read the text that follows the case without skipping first to the answers at the end of each chapter. Then go back to the question and see whether you can answer it a little more comprehensively. Finally, check the answers. This is our version of the Socratic Method, a mode of teaching that we favor.

Mnemonics

Scattered throughout the book are mnemonics (memory aids; from the Greek *mnēmon*, mindful) which we have invented over the years. They can be used as teaching devices or in clinical settings to recall the list of symptoms or characteristics of the topic at hand.

Appendix A: Glossary of terms

We have attempted to define all terms that you will encounter in this book. Additionally, there are terms in the appendix that are not in the chapters. We figured that during your clinical rounds or classes you might encounter additional terms relevant to understanding psychosis and schizophrenia.

Appendix B: Medications commonly used in treating schizophrenia

Refer to this appendix when you need a quick overview.

Appendixes C and D: Bibliography and sources of help and information

This is where you will find a listing of books and references, organizations, and websites that can further your education and prove useful to patients and families. Remember that such a listing is necessarily partial and current only to the date of publishing.

Feedback

We would be pleased to hear from you at our website: www.schizophrenia-primer.com where you can post opinions, suggestions, errors of fact or judgment, and new information for future students.

The poetry is by Ravinder Reddy and the cartoons are by Matcheri Keshavan. We like aphorisms and quotations. Here is one of our favorite quotations about books:

The worth of a book is to be measured by what you can carry away from it.
James Bryce (1838–1922)

We hope that *Schizophrenia: A Practical Primer* serves its purpose.

Ravinder Reddy
Matcheri Keshavan

chapter 1

What is and is not schizophrenia?

Stop, Go, To and fro
It hurts, damn it, it hurts so
But don't you come near
You, who burned my brain clear

The term 'schizophrenia' was coined almost a century ago by the Swiss psychiatrist Eugen Bleuler. He wanted to capture the notion of a 'fractured' or 'shattered' mind. Because of a long tradition of scientific terms being derived from Greek, Bleuler combined σχιζω (*schizo*, split or divide) and φρενος (*phrenos*, mind) to arrive at schizophrenia.

Before considering what schizophrenia is, it is important to grasp the concept of psychosis, because it is central to the definition of schizophrenia.

The definition of psychosis varies depending on where you seek it. It is not uncommon for psychosis to be defined as a mental disorder. Rather than being a *disorder*, psychosis is best thought of as a clinical state, analogous to having fever. Just as fever reflects ongoing disturbance of temperature regulation, psychosis reflects brain dysfunction. Fever has many causes, and so does psychosis.

> Psychosis is a state characterized by loss of contact with reality, with a variety of manifestations – false beliefs (delusions), false perceptions (hallucinations), irrational thinking and behaviors.

All formal definitions of schizophrenia (two of which are widely used – Diagnostic and Statistical Manual (DSM) and International Classification of Diseases (ICD)) require the presence of psychosis. However, it is important to remember that the presence of psychosis *alone* does not make it schizophrenia. In other words, schizophrenia is a form of psychosis, but not all psychosis is schizophrenia.

Psychosis is seen in a wide variety of disorders. In some, it is integral to the definition of the disorder. In other conditions, psychosis is neither essential to the diagnosis nor is it necessarily present. There is a long list of non-psychiatric conditions (see Chapter 5) in which psychosis can occur. Table 1.1 gives a list of *psychiatric* disorders in which psychosis occurs.

Table 1.1 Psychiatric disorders associated with psychosis

Disorders in which psychosis is integral to the definition	*Psychosis is observed but not essential to define the disorder*
Schizophrenia	Delirium
Schizophreniform Disorder	Dementia
Brief Psychotic Disorder	Mood disorders
Schizoaffective Disorder	Borderline Personality Disorder
Delusional Disorder	Substance-related disorders
Shared Psychotic Disorder	

The sufferers

Approximately 50 million individuals worldwide suffer from schizophrenia. In the USA, there are approximately 2.2 million individuals diagnosed with schizophrenia. It is estimated that about one-third or more individuals with schizophrenia have not been in treatment for the past 12 months.

The direct costs of the illness, that is, the cost of caring for these patients, in the USA alone exceeds $19 billion per year. The indirect costs, such as productivity, may well exceed $60 billion per year.

Of approximately 600 000 homeless individuals in the USA, a third are severely mentally ill, with as many as half of them suffering from schizophrenia.

The longevity of persons with schizophrenia is reduced by an average of 10 years, due to both unnatural and natural causes (such as cardiovascular diseases). Ten per cent of patients with schizophrenia commit suicide.

The myths

Myths are a means of understanding the world and our place in it. Schizophrenia, like epilepsy before it, has been viewed as being 'un-understandable', and therefore evokes myths as explanations. Myths, like ignorance, can lead to troubling consequences – stigma and denial. The best way to contend with ignorance is by education.

We suggest asking patients and their families about *their* understanding of schizophrenia, so that any mythology of schizophrenia they might subscribe to can be addressed directly. In all instances it is our *duty* to provide education about the current understanding of schizophrenia and its treatment. Some of the common myths encountered and your potential responses are listed in Table 1.2.

The stigma of schizophrenia

I take my pills
I even pay my bills
But don't you ask me to luv ya
You SOB, calling me a psycha

Stigma is largely a consequence of not understanding the nature of schizophrenia. The 'un-understandable', like the unknown, can be fearful. It is human nature to fight or flee fearful situations. The consequences of such actions against patients with schizophrenia, unfortunately, are life altering.

Schizophrenia, like 'crazy' or 'mad', evokes a variety of images, either naïve or pejorative, usually both. Patients with schizophrenia were (in some cases still are) treated like lepers. Hopefully, as we move towards a more enlightened view of schizophrenia – a disabling disease of the brain – the more tolerant society will become of these unfortunate individuals.

Today, we understand schizophrenia to mean an illness that impairs thinking, feeling, and the ability to accurately perceive reality – it affects the

Table 1.2 A sampling of common and widespread myths about schizophrenia

Common and widespread myth	Your response
It is 'split personality'	A very common misunderstanding due to the origin of the word (*schizo*, split + *phrenia*, mind). It is not multiple personality disorder
It only runs in families	It is true that there is genetic transmission of schizophrenia, but a substantial number of patients have no family history of the illness
Patients are violent or dangerous	No more than others in the general population. There are patients who act aggressively as a result of the psychosis, particularly paranoia
There is no effective treatment	There are very effective treatments, although a great deal of variation exists in response to treatment
It is due to bad parenting, especially the mothers	The so-called *schizophrenogenic* mother was held responsible. There is no evidence that bad parenting causes schizophrenia; bad parenting just adds to the patient's misery
It is due to drug abuse	Drug abuse is very common in patients with schizophrenia, particularly at the onset of illness. The evidence is not entirely clear about drug abuse causing or precipitating schizophrenia. We know that it can interfere with treatment
It is their fault	It is not the fault of the patient. No one chooses to have schizophrenia!

Children don't get it	Although schizophrenia typically emerges in late adolescence and adulthood, it can appear in early life (childhood schizophrenia). Treatment is similar to adult schizophrenia
Marriage 'cures' schizophrenia	In some cultures it is believed that marriage cures schizophrenia. There is no evidence for this. While the possibility exists that marriage may have beneficial effects (due to a caring partner), it can just as easily be problematic
Evil spirits cause schizophrenia	In some communities there are strong beliefs about supernatural causes of suffering. It is best to work with, rather than against, these beliefs. Our approach is to suggest that conventional (modern) treatments can work alongside efforts to cast off evil spirits, so that patients are not forced to choose the non-medical approach
Patients are 'possessed'	This is analogous to 'evil spirits' but not identical. Possession can occur with 'spirits' of all sorts – good, bad or neutral. The same approach as above is recommended
Past misdeeds cause it	In cultures where belief of past lives exists, present suffering is attributed to past actions, usually 'sins'. Our approach is to suggest to patients and their families that the best we can do is rectify the suffering in the present
Only rituals cure schizophrenia	This is one of the most challenging myths to deal with because individuals and families who utilize traditional rituals will try these first before seeking medical help. This results in longer duration of untreated psychosis which is a risk factor for poor outcome
A spell has been cast	Similar to other supernatural attributions for schizophrenia, being under a spell is quite common. In addition to problems of engaging patients into treatment, there is a risk that patients or their families may retaliate against the spell-caster, if known

Table 1.2 continued

They are stupid	The thinking disturbance of schizophrenia can be mistaken for 'stupidity'
A person with schizophrenia is blessed and holy	The only advantage with this myth is that the patient tends not to be mistreated. However, there can be reluctance in seeking treatment. Patients don't want to run the risk of losing the numinous experience
It is treatment for life	Once diagnosis of schizophrenia is made with certainty, treatment may continue for a lifetime. However, if patients remain symptom-free for long periods of time, lowering the dose of medications may be tried
Schizophrenia is just a myth, a label	There are sociological and political reasons why schizophrenia is considered by some as an invention of the psychiatric establishment for its own (nefarious?) purposes. No doubt that the fear of being labeled schizophrenic is frightening to all. The consequences, however, of accepting schizophrenic as simply a myth are not inconsequential, mostly for those individuals who suffer from its effects
	There is no such condition as schizophrenia, but the label is a social fact and the social fact a political event. R. D. Laing (1927–1989)
	However, we agree with what Dr Laing once said: *Schizophrenia cannot be understood without understanding despair.*

whole individual. It can cause ANGUISH (Table 1.3) and cripple the individual, deeply affect his or her family, and deprive the community of a fully participant member.

Table 1.3. Consequences of stigma (ANGUISH)

Alone	Patients, as well as their families suffer in silence. This can lead to social isolation. There is also a tendency to 'cover up' the illness
Negative experiences	Patients will suffer all sorts of negative experiences. Name-calling, inability to complete school work, no job offers, losing friends, being asked to leave business establishments, and so on
Guilt and shame	These feelings are commonly experienced by patients and families, leading to distorted perceptions of self
Untreated illness duration	Increased duration of untreated illness is a strong predictor of poor outcome
Incarceration	Because of untreated illness, disturbing behaviors can result in legal trouble, and such individuals can be lost to psychiatric care for long periods of time. Increasingly, enlightened legal systems are recognizing mental illness in their inmates and providing treatment
Substance abuse	Illicit drugs and alcohol are often used to deal with the psychological pain, leading to its own set of problems
Health worsens	Avoidance or lack of healthcare access also contributes to poorer physical health

Summary
- The term 'schizophrenia' was coined to capture the notion of a 'fractured' or 'shattered' mind, not *split mind*.
- Psychosis is a state characterized by loss of contact with reality.
- Not all psychosis is schizophrenia, but schizophrenia is a form of psychosis.
- Approximately 50 million individuals worldwide suffer from schizophrenia. The suffering and economic costs are enormous.

- Many homeless individuals are mentally ill, about half of whom suffer from schizophrenia.
- Stigma has powerful negative effects and should be combated.
- Myths about schizophrenia are numerous and found worldwide. They are associated with stigma and denial of illness. Stigma should be combated vigorously by education.

chapter 2

Assessment of schizophrenia

Can't line up straight lines
Can't tell forest from pines
Street corners with no bloody signs

Birds, turds, brain matters
Hear them little patters?
Heck, my mind's all a tatters!

Before assessing patients who have schizophrenia or similar conditions, it is useful to take a moment to think about one's perceptions about individuals with psychosis.

You observe a shabbily dressed young man at the street corner, waving at passing cars, and apparently talking to himself. He sees you watching him, catches your eye, and begins to move towards you. You hastily turn your eyes and walk away.

Q2.1 Is this person:

a) angry

b) lonely

c) psychotic

d) manic

e) an addict

You thought he was dangerous because:

a) he was acting abnormally

b) he must be dangerous *because* his behavior would indicate so

General principles

Do you feel depressed? Do you feel anxious?
These are straightforward questions likely to get straightforward responses.

Do you feel psychotic? Are you experiencing schizophrenia?
While these are straightforward questions they do not work well.

Assessing the clinical state of patients with schizophrenia can be challenging, unintuitive and frustrating. This is due to the nature of the illness. Communicating with patients with schizophrenia can be hampered by the presence of thinking difficulties, delusions, and hallucinations. This is true, in fact, for all disorders that are accompanied by psychotic phenomena.

Interviewing a patient with psychosis can be an anxiety-provoking experience for the novice. Patients are frequently uncooperative or outright hostile. Alternatively, they may be cooperative but unable to communicate effectively.

Most importantly, remember that the person in front of you is *not* a 'psychotic' or a 'schizophrenic', however convenient these labels might be; rather, you are interacting with an individual suffering *from* a psychotic disorder, just as you or I might suffer from cancer or mental retardation. (We wouldn't like to be referred to as cancerous or retarded!) Remembering this will ease the fear and frustrations one may experience while interviewing patients with psychosis.

Observe experienced clinicians interviewing patients with psychotic disorders. If possible, interview patients *without* psychosis a few times prior to interviewing patients with psychosis. You will feel more practiced in your interview method.

While interviewing *any* patient it is important to:

- be non-judgmental
- be patient
- use vocabulary familiar to the patient (no jargon)
- inquire about the details of the history
- offer hope and support.

EMPATHY is a quality whereby it is perceived by the patient that the interviewer has a genuine appreciation of his or her distress. Empathy cannot be 'manufactured' or pretended for any length of time. The best expression of empathy is genuine caring about the patient and his or her problems by sensitive and detailed understanding of the issues. No amount of 'empathetic noises' such as, 'That must have been terrible' or 'I understand' can substitute for genuine empathy. While *sympathy* has a role in interviewing, overdoing it is counterproductive.

HUMOR can be a useful tool in assessing mental state or facilitating therapeutic alliance, but there is significant risk of a misfired moment during an interview – or worse, a joke or humorous turn of phrase being misconstrued. Smiling at something humorous said or done by the patient is fine if it was intended to be funny, but beware of uncontrolled guffaws!

Interviewing an individual suspected of experiencing psychosis

Allow the patient to tell his or her story. If the patient is silent or unwilling to talk, begin by asking about their understanding of why they are at this place now or about the trip to the clinic or hospital, or about their living situation.

A lot can be learned by listening to the initial verbalization. The flow of speech can reveal thinking disturbances. (Is the thinking linear or disordered?) The construction of the speech can betray aphasias or disturbances in logic. Delusions can become apparent by the content of the speech (statements about being spied upon by police cameras, for example).

Think of the interview as a series of OLA ('hello' in Spanish):

Observe behavior
Listen especially to spontaneous verbalization
Ask open-ended, leading or follow-up questions as required.

Even if the focus of the interview is psychosis, make sure to ask about other conditions to ensure a comprehensive diagnostic assessment.

How much to ask and when?

All interviews are conducted within a set of constraints:

- time (the amount of time practicably available)
- location (emergency room, inpatient unit, outpatient service)
- patient's capacity to communicate (verbal, guarded, rambling, or mute)
- dangerousness of patient's behavior (aggressive, violent, acutely suicidal).

Your task is to discover the most salient information relevant to the predicted outcome of the interview. If you anticipate hospitalization, consider what kinds of information you'd like to have immediately and what information can be gathered later. For example, for an acutely suicidal patient, gathering family history may not be the most important task at this time. If the patient is seeking transfer of outpatient care, likely you'll want specific information to assure smooth transition of care, such as reason for transfer, recent course of treatment, and so forth.

That said, at a minimum you need to determine whether the patient is dangerous to self or others (reviewed in Chapter 14), is using illicit substances, is compliant with treatment if previously treated, and whether there is any ongoing medical problem.

JB is being seen at a busy emergency service because of incessant suicidal thoughts. You have no previous medical notes because she has not been seen at this hospital before.

Q2.2 Which of the following questions are least important at this time?
a) Have you attempted suicide before?
b) Is anyone in your family depressed?
c) Are you hearing voices commanding you?
d) Are you taking any medicine?
e) Were you subject to abuse growing up?
f) Do you live alone?

AK, a 17-year-old, comes to the clinic accompanied by his mother. She made this first appointment because of her concerns that AK is isolating himself, sometimes laughs for no apparent reason, his mood is erratic and he stays up all night.

Q2.3 What information will you want to gather before the end of a 45-minute evaluation?
   a) Is AK using drugs?
   b) Is AK sexually active?
   c) Does anyone in the family have schizophrenia?
   d) Is AK experiencing hallucinations?
   e) How are the parents getting along?
   f) How is AK doing in school?

Manner of questioning

There are many techniques and stratagems that are available in the service of eliciting information. With practice one can learn how and when to apply them appropriately. Conducting lots of interviews and watching experienced interviewers can greatly enhance one's skills. The basic types of question are:

- open-ended (*how have you been feeling?*)
- leading (*you've been feeling poorly lately, haven't you?*)
- closed-ended (*are you depressed?*)

Patients with schizophrenia often require closed-ended and leading questions to move the interview along and to gather information. This is usually due to cognitive deficits and negative symptoms. Paranoia also can significantly impair the flow of the information.

The interviewer asks a patient the following questions:

1) *Are you paranoid?*
2) *What are you bothered by?*
3) *Are you perhaps imagining all this?*
4) *Have you ever behaved in an unusual manner?*

Q2.4 Match the number to the letter:
   a) Appropriate in the right context
   b) Inappropriate
   c) Open-ended
   d) Leading

AGREE WITH A DELUSION OR CHALLENGE IT?

A rule of thumb is to agree with the patient with the same degree of firmness with which the patient holds the delusions. Weakly held delusions can be challenged, but strongly held delusions are best addressed by passive acknowledgment, but neither challenging nor agreeing with them. A common fear is that agreeing to a delusion will further entrench the delusional thinking. Recall the definition of a delusion – a belief that is held in spite of evidence to the contrary. Remember, though, that you do not have to condone the content of the delusions.

Imagining psychosis

Unlike depression or anxiety, our ability to genuinely understand psychotic phenomena is limited. However, it is important to try to *imagine* what a psychotic experience may be like for the patient. Put yourself in their 'shoes': imagine what it might feel like to be spied upon constantly or to have persecutory voices tormenting you. Such an exercise will not only help you to phrase questions in helpful ways and assist patients to articulate their experiences, but also engender empathy. It is quite common for patients with schizophrenia to have difficulty in describing psychotic phenomena or not be fully forthcoming about the effect of psychosis on their lives. One of our favorite phrases during interviewing is, 'I wonder . . .'

I wonder whether you keep a weapon nearby in case the people trying to hurt you or break into your apartment.

I wonder whether the voices that bother you say really awful things about you, things that you would never reveal to anyone.

I wonder whether you feel like you don't fit in because of your illness.

If I thought that others could read my mind, I might be forced to stop having thoughts that they could pick up. I wonder if you feel that way.

We have found this approach to be very useful in getting patients to talk about the distress they experience. We do refrain from using this approach in patients who are experiencing severe thought broadcasting (i.e. the sense that others can read one's thoughts) because they experience these questions as validation of their psychotic experience, which can lead to further distress.

Mental status examination

The mental status examination (MSE), analogous to a physical examination, is a process by which the clinician investigates mental functioning. The history and MSE constitute a psychiatric examination. Typically the MSE follows obtaining a comprehensive history. In reality the MSE occurs in conjunction with obtaining the history, beginning the moment the patient is seen, even before any conversation occurs. A proper mental status exam will have the following components we call the 'A-to-J' of MSE:

- Appearance
- Behavior
- Conversation – to listen to the *form* of thinking
- Delusions - to listen to the *content* of thinking
- Emotions – mood and affect
- Faculties - higher faculties such as attention and orientation
- General intelligence
- Hallucinations
- Insight
- Judgment

Assessing the major components of psychosis

Psychosis is most commonly established by the presence of delusions, hallucinations, or thought disorder. Additionally, patients present with emotional, behavioral, cognitive, and neurological disturbances that accompany psychosis.

Mr O reports he is concerned that his wife has been having an affair for the past several months. He thinks this because she doesn't answer her phone at work and returns home smelling 'funny'.

Q2.5 Is the patient paranoid? If so, how do you know this?

Delusions

Delusions are false beliefs. More properly, a delusion is a fixed, false belief that is held in spite of evidence to the contrary, is at odds with the community's cultural and religious beliefs, is inconsistent with the level of education of the patient, and can be patently absurd. Overvalued ideas are beliefs which are less firmly held than delusions and tend to be less absurd; they are more easily challenged.

Delusions can be well organized with ideas connected to each other (systematized delusions), or non-systematized and fragmented. It is not uncommon for patients also to have intense preoccupation with esoteric and vague ideas about philosophical, religious, or psychological themes. Hypochondriacal thinking about unlikely and bizarre medical conditions may also occur. Delusions can be about any sort of idea, but the most common ones are listed in Table 2.1.

Table 2.1 Common delusions

Term	Observations in patients
Paranoid	Feeling persecuted; feeling taken advantage of; conspiracy of harm or spying; messages in innocuous events
Grandiose	Unique or superior abilities; special powers; superior personage
Somatic	Sense that something is uniquely wrong with the body that has not been or cannot be detected by others
Erotomanic	Convinced that someone famous, beautiful, rich or otherwise beyond reach is in love with the patient; also known as Clérambault's syndrome
Jealous	Sometimes referred to as the Othello syndrome; the patient is convinced that a spouse or partner is cheating
Thought insertion	Belief or experience that outside forces or entities place thoughts into one's mind
Thought broadcasting	Belief or experience that one's thoughts are broadcast to the external world and may be 'read' by others
Referential thinking	Also called ideas of reference, wherein the individual interprets common events as having personal relevance (e.g. messages from the TV or songs, or innocuous gestures signifying specific codes).
Delusions of passivity	A sense that the mind or body is being controlled or interfered with by external forces or persons

How do we discover that a patient is delusional?

Not by asking, *'are you delusional?'* or, *'do you have unusual ideas?'* Delusional thinking can be picked up by listening to what the patient is expressing, particularly their concerns. Not infrequently, though, patients will not divulge their thoughts spontaneously. In such cases, it is useful to ask rather directly: in other words, **OLA** (observe, listen, ask).

By listening carefully, one can get clues about delusional thinking. The trick is to follow up with questions that can sensitively probe further.

> **Patient:** I had to take two buses to get here. You'd think that they'd at least let me sit down. By the way, can I have bus tokens to get back home? I used my last tokens on that stupid bus.

Q2.6 Is there anything worthwhile following up in this statement?

Hallucinations

Hallucinations are false perceptions (Table 2.2). These occur in the *absence* of a stimulus, and can involve any of the bodily sensations (seeing, hearing, smelling, tasting and feeling). **Illusions**, on the other hand, are *misperceptions* of actual stimuli. Illusions are not typically considered psychotic phenomena, although they are commonly experienced by patients with schizophrenia. The most common hallucination in schizophrenia is auditory (70–80% of patients). The presence alone of visual or olfactory hallucinations should raise suspicion of underlying medical or neurological disorder.

How do we discover that a patient is experiencing hallucinations?

Unlike in the case of delusions, it is usually a good idea to ask directly about hallucinations if not already divulged by the patient. For example, one could ask:

Have you ever heard sounds or voices in your head or even from the outside that you couldn't quite figure out? Have you ever heard voices that other people didn't hear?

Have you seen things or had visions that didn't quite fit with what was going on at the time? Did you ever see things or people that others couldn't see at the same time?

What about feeling or sensations in your body that were different from your usual experiences?

Have you smelled or tasted anything unusual – it could be nice, like perfume or bad, like burning flesh, or some taste like metal?

Table 2.2 Hallucinations

Term	Observations in patients
Auditory	Hearing sounds; unintelligible whispers; single words (such as a name) or sentences; single or multiple familiar or unfamiliar voices; comments on patient's actions; conversing among speakers; voices commanding actions, including harm to others and self, or sexual acts (command hallucinations); varying loudness; commonly worse when alone; patients talking to self usually in response to auditor hallucinations
Visual	Seeing shadows at the corner of eye; ghost-like images; natural and unnatural objects; partial or complete images of known or unknown persons; complete scenes of events, commonly disturbing images
Somatosensory	Transient sensations of pain, electricity or movement; sensations that body parts are moving, including the brain; shrinking of body parts; alterations in shape, color or texture of body parts, including skin
Olfactory	Usually unpleasant smells (such as feces, burning rubber or flesh), but occasionally pleasant smells like perfume or fruits
Gustatory	Unusual tastes, particularly metallic or salty

Thought disturbance

The structure of thinking is reflected in speech and writing, and behavior. Disordered thinking is common in schizophrenia and takes on many forms. The end result of thought disorder is impaired communication (see below).

Clinician: *How are you feeling today?*

Patient: *Fine, doc. But these humanoids really suck. The universe is particulate. I just wish they'd stop squeezing my intestines. How are you doc?* (Smiling)

Q2.7   Describe the thought process here.

Thought disturbance can be subtle, so as not to interfere with most communication or so severe that speech is unintelligible. Common types of thought
disorder are listed in Table 2.3.

Table 2.3 Thought process disturbance

Term	Observations in patients
Circumstantiality	Speech is over-inclusive with detail; thoughts start off linearly, but then wander off for a while, returning later to the original point. In order to detect circumstantiality it is important to allow the patient to speak for a period of time before interrupting
Tangentiality	Thoughts start off linearly, but quickly veer off into unrelated areas without returning to the original point. When interrupted, patients tend to ask what the question was in the first place
Loose associations	There is an apparent disconnection between one thought (usually a sentence) and the next. An indication that loosening of associations is occurring is when the interviewer is unable to follow the train of thought ('huh?'). When severe, speech becomes incomprehensible
Thought blocking	In mid-sentence the patient appears to have lost the train of thought. However, you need to ascertain whether the patient actually 'lost' the thought – true thought blocking – or was distracted by competing thoughts
Flight of ideas	This represents a combination of thought disorders. Here a fairly complete idea is followed by another idea with only a tenuous or no connection between these thoughts. One experiences it as a zigzagging through conversation
Neologism	Coining of new terms with idiosyncratic meanings (e.g. 'flushistic')
Perseveration	Persistent repetition of a response to new and unrelated stimuli
Verbigeration	Persistent repetition of words or phrases (e.g. 'I was going the corrected way. They hadn't corrected the signs, and now I was lost and had to get corrected directions.')
Word salad	Complete lack of meaningful connections between words (e.g. 'seeing blasts tin hatched flour all along'). This thought disturbance is quite rare

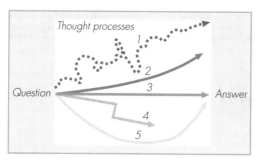

Q2.8 Match the number with the letter:

a) Linear thinking

b) Flight of ideas

c) Loss of associations

d) Circumstantiality

e) Tangentiality

How do we discover that a patient has a thought disorder?

Unlike assessment of hallucinations or delusions, thought disorder is best detected by listening. Open-ended questions are the most effective for eliciting thought disorder.

To determine *past* thought disorder, in the absence of medical records or corroborative information, it is useful to ask the patient something like:

Was there a time in the past when people complained that they couldn't quite follow what you were saying?

Have you ever noticed that your thinking was muddled?

Did you ever notice that, in the middle of a thought, it just sort of disappeared and you couldn't recall it?

Negative symptoms

In addition to psychosis, patients with schizophrenia commonly exhibit negative symptoms. These are a constellation of signs and symptoms that are characterized by diminution or loss of functioning (Table 2.4). This is in contrast to **positive symptoms** (hallucinations and delusions) which reflect augmentation or addition of functioning.

Negative symptoms are classified as *primary* (due to the illness itself) or *secondary* (consequence of the illness and its treatment). The importance of this distinction lies in their treatment (see Chapter 9). Negative symptoms can be especially bothersome to patients and are often resistant to treatment (Figure 2.1).

Table 2.4 Negative symptoms

Term	Function affected	Observations in patients
Alogia	Fluency of speech	Reduced quantity of speech; brief answers to questions; monosyllabic responses, such as 'yes' or 'no'
Affective blunting	Emotional expression	Reduced range of facial and body movement classified as restricted, blunted, and flat (mild, moderate and severe, respectively); sitting in a chair with little movement
Avolition	Volition and drive	Frequently confused with laziness because patients have difficulty initiating or following through tasks; inability to plan for the future
Anhedonia	Hedonic capacity	Inability to enjoy activities previously found pleasurable, including intimacy; performing tasks in a mechanical, bored manner; staring at the television for hours with no indication of enjoyment
Asociality	Social interactions	Tendency to isolate

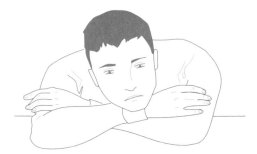

Figure 2.1 Patient with negative symptoms. Note the mask face, and social withdrawal.

Disturbances of emotion

Patients with schizophrenia present with a variety of emotional states – anxiety, perplexity, elation, or depression. Expansive mood may present as ecstasy or exaltation (sometimes confused with religious experiences). Inappropriate affect, which is the disconnection between the display of emotion and the thought and speech content, is quite common (e.g. the patient may grin while describing a sad event, or burst into tears while describing an amusing situation).

Behavioral disturbances

Schizophrenia patients frequently manifest psychomotor and behavioral abnormalities (Table 2.5). These behaviors are not necessarily a consequence of underlying delusions or hallucinations.

Cognitive abnormalities

There has been increasing focus on cognition (higher intellectual functioning including awareness, perception, reasoning, memory, and problem solving) in schizophrenia. Advances in cognitive neurosciences have significantly bolstered our understanding of the nature of cognitive disturbances in schizophrenia and treatments are being developed to remediate these deficits (Table 2.6).

Table 2.5 Behavioral disturbances

Term	Observations in patients
Posturing	The assumption of odd postures
Mannerisms	Goal-directed behaviors carried out in an odd or stilted fashion
Stereotypies	Non-purposeful and uniformly repetitive motions, such as tapping and rocking
Echopraxia	The repetitive imitation of movements performed by others
Echolalia	The repetitive imitation of words or statements made by others
Catatonia	There are two forms of catatonia – stuporous and excited. Catatonic stupor presents as immobility, posturing (waxy flexibility), mutism and negativity. Catatonic excitement presents as excited and aimless motor activity

Table 2.6 Cognitive deficits

Domain	Function affected	Observations in patients
Attention	Ability to focus on specific aspects of the environment while excluding others	Distractibility; inability to stay on task
Perception and recognition		Missing the point of conversation
Memory	Working memory, verbal learning and memory, visual learning and memory	Impaired recall of facts, stories, ideas
Language	Perception, processing and production of language	Impaired syntax, vocabulary, and speech output
Executive functions	Problem solving, planning, reasoning	Deficits in planning, sequencing of actions, concept formation, mental set shifting, and selective attention

Neurological abnormalities

Patients with schizophrenia can have subtle neurologic disturbances, referred to as 'soft signs,' which consist of disturbances in **motor coordination** (gait, balance, coordination, and muscle tone), **sensory integration** (graphesthesia, stereognosis, and proprioception) and **primitive reflexes** (such as the palmomental, grasp, and snout reflexes). While these findings clearly substantiate the biological basis of schizophrenia, they do not necessarily help us with the diagnosis of this illness.

Summary (see also Table 2.7)

- Interviewing a patient with psychosis can be an anxiety-provoking experience for the novice. Remembering the person in front of you is *not* a 'psychotic', but an individual suffering *from* a psychotic disorder, will ease the fear and frustration.
- While interviewing it is important to remain nonjudgmental, patient, plain-speaking (no jargon), and offer hope and support.

- When interviewing an individual suspected of experiencing psychosis, allow the patient to tell his or her story.
- A lot can be learned by listening to the initial speech; thinking disturbances can be revealed and delusions may become apparent by the content of the speech.

Table 2.7 Assessment strategies

The issue	What to do
Uncovering delusions	First listen; the manner and content of the verbalizations will offer many clues to delusional thinking; then probe sensitively about the details of the delusions, and their effect on the patient's life; do not challenge the delusion
Uncovering hallucinations	Observe first; does the patient appear distracted, as if attending to some inner voices or visions; is the patient mumbling or talking to self aloud? If required, ask directly about hallucinatory experiences
Uncovering thought disorder	Listen; don't interrupt prematurely; ensure that the patient understood the question correctly so as not to mislabel the response!
Negative symptoms	Observe facial expression, particularly in response to material that could elicit feelings; note whether gestures are used and the body's posture; ask about pleasurable activities; ask about future plans; ask about the week's activities
The angry patient	There are many reasons why patients present with anger – there may be situational reasons, such as being brought in against their will, or due to underlying paranoia or irritability. The first order of business is to ensure everyone's safety. A patient who is helped to feel safe is less likely to remain angry or act out aggressively. Acknowledge the patient's anger. Enquire whether the patient would like food or water. If the patient begins to shout, it is alright to state that the shouting is interfering with your ability to help the patient.
The paranoid patient	The issue is one of trusting the interviewer. Sometimes it helps to ally with the (acceptable) delusions to gain trust. The 'us against them' approach is useful only so long as the patient doesn't start to incorporate the interviewer into the delusional system!

- The interview is a process of observation, listening and asking questions.
- All interviews are conducted within a set of constraints, but at a minimum determine whether the patient is dangerous to self or others, is using illicit substances, is compliant with treatment, and whether there are any ongoing medical problems.

ANSWERS

Q2.1 Any unusual behavior in our environment gets our attention - we are a curious species! However, it is also our nature to determine whether an unusual event is a threat. The individual at the street corner comes to our attention primarily because of the set of behaviors that he or she displays. Any one of those behaviors individually would not necessarily attract our attention. However, the juxtaposition of those behaviors is suggestive of abnormality and, in our minds, irrationality and dangerousness. Thus, when that individual begins to approach you, fear (of the unknown) takes over.

Q2.2 The questions you want to ask for certain:

Have you attempted suicide before? Past suicide attempts are a strong predictor of suicide.
Are you hearing voices commanding you? Auditory hallucinations commanding harm to self can be incessant and patients can 'give in' to the voices.
Are you taking any medicine? This can tell you about whether the patient is in treatment, level of compliance, whether there is access to medications with overdose potential.
Do you live alone? Living alone is a risk factor for suicide.

These questions can generally wait for later:

Is anyone in your family depressed? This gives you an indication that depression may be familial. It will not necessarily help with estimating current risk of suicide; instead ask about suicide in relatives, a better predictor of suicide.
Were you subject to abuse growing up? This is an important issue that may or may not be associated with current suicide risk. It certainly would be important to address in ongoing therapy.

Q2.3 The initial interview is to arrive at a working diagnosis and management plan. The following questions will be necessary to acomplish this:

Is AK using drugs? Practically all substances of abuse are associated with altered behavior, including psychosis.

Is AK experiencing hallucinations? Hallucinations are a common psychotic phenomenon, particularly in schizophrenia.

How is AK doing in school? This can be a valuable indicator of how AK's functioning has been affected by recent changes in behavior. Decline in functioning is one of the criteria for diagnostic threshold for many psychiatric disorders, including schizophrenia.

Does anyone in the family have schizophrenia? If there is a family history of schizophrenia, it allows estimation of risk of a psychotic disorder, but does not provide diagnostic certainty.

These questions can wait till later meetings:

How are mother and father getting along? Many disorders, including schizophrenia, are precipitated by psychosocial stressors. However, the assessment of family dynamics may not be important at this stage of assessment. Family involvement can be positive for patients while over-involvement can have detrimental effects.

Is AK sexually active? This may be indicative of AK's social skills, ability to establish relationships, but is not helpful in deriving a diagnosis.

Q2.4 1) *Are you paranoid?* b) Inappropriate
2) *What are you bothered by?* c) Open-ended
3) *Are you perhaps imagining all this?* a) Appropriate in the right context
4) *Have you ever behaved in an unusual manner?* d) Leading

Q2.5 Mr. O is clearly suspicious of his wife's fidelity. More questions need to be asked to determine if his concerns are plausible or are based on 'flimsy' evidence. If the evidence presented appears implausible, then a delusion should be suspected. However, it is necessary to challenge Mr. O's assumptions in order to determine how firmly these beliefs are held. For example, one could ask, 'is it possible, for sake of argument, that you are mistaken about your wife actually having an affair?' Not allowing for even the possibility that he may be mistaken strengthens the case for the presence of a delusion (of jealously).

Q2.6 It would be useful to inquire about the events on the bus. The patient is clearly upset about something he experienced on the 'stupid' bus.

Q2.7 The patient is exhibiting loss of association, neologism ('the universe is particulate'), and inappropriate affect.

Q2.8 1) c) Loss of associations
2) e) Tangentiality
3) a) Linear thinking
4) b) Flight of ideas
5) d) Circumstantiality

chapter 3

Non-illness related factors affecting assessment

What 'sick' in general may mean depends less on a doctor's judgment than on the judgment of the patient and the prevailing conceptions of the contemporary culture ... With psychic illness [this] is very much so. The same psychic state will bring the one individual to he psychiatrist as a sick person while it will take another to the confessional as one suffering from sin and guilt.

Karl Jaspers (1883–1969)

A variety of factors can affect the clinical presentation and treatment of schizophrenia. These factors, which are independent of the illness, can modify the clinical picture as well as the outcome of treatment. Thus, assessment and treatment planning must take these factors into account

One view is that all peoples of the world are essentially the same biologically, particularly with regard to brain functioning (*universalism*). Thus, with the exception of a few minor differences, schizophrenia essentially ought to be the same across the world. This view was supported by landmark studies by the World Health Organization (WHO) in the 1970s. The International Pilot Study of Schizophrenia found that the clinical presentation of schizophrenia in the 10 countries was essentially the same (Figure 3.1).

On the other hand, there has been increasing appreciation that culture itself can shape individual worldview and perceptions and affect illness presentation, attribution of meaning of the illness, and even the outcome of treatment. The same WHO studies that noted similarities in the clinical presentation of schizophrenia across continents found significant differences in treatment outcome. Contrary to expectations, patients from developing countries like India and Nigeria fared better than patients from the USA and UK. The difference in outcome may be attributed to variations in social factors, treatment response, or diet. Thus, there are relative differences among peoples (*relativism*) that need to be taken into account during clinical assessment and treatment.

RC is a 31-year-old woman of Asian origin who lives alone; she recently moved to the UK for postgraduate studies. She is referred to the clinic because of her insistent complaints that the male professors are failing her because she is smarter than them. She is certain because she hears them talking about her brilliance and her 'foreign' looks.

Q3.1 Which of the following factors may be important in RC's presentation? Why?
a) Educational achievements
b) Ethnicity
c) Immigration
d) Culture
e) Age

An individual's 'LEGACIE' can significantly influence the risk of developing schizophrenia, the expression of the illness, the treatment response and long-term clinical outcome. There is a long list of biological and non-biological factors that have a role in schizophrenia. Discussed below are factors that have been identified as important, some of which have been quite well researched.

Location
Ethnicity
Gender
Age
Culture
Immigration
Environment

MA is a 27-year-old individual with a full-time job, who presents with acute-onset paranoia, auditory hallucinations, depressed mood and confusion. MA is treated with 2 mg risperidone, with almost complete resolution of symptoms and no negative symptoms. MA did well in school with no notable social difficulties.

Q3.2 Do you think MA is male or female?
Why?

Gender

Sex and gender, while seemingly the same terms, are not identical. Sex denotes biological male or female (*what you are born with*), while gender is maleness and femaleness, the sum of psychosocial development (*what you are given and become*). There are several important distinctions between men and women with schizophrenia regarding the clinical picture, treatment response, and long-term outcome. It has been theorized that these differences may be due to biological (e.g. estrogen) and environmental factors (e.g. better socialization in women) (Table 3.1).

Table 3.1 Gender differences

	Women	Men
Age at onset of illness	Onset 5 years later than men. However, late-onset schizophrenia is more common in women	Earlier onset, in late teens and early adulthood
Onset of illness	Rapid onset	Insidious onset
Clinical presentation	More commonly present with depressed mood, paranoia, fewer negative symptoms, and better functioning while ill	More negative symptoms
Treatment response	More rapid and complete response to initial treatment. However, women are more likely to have side effects	Relatively a more gradual response, with persistence of symptoms, particularly negative symptoms
Long-term outcome	Better than men	Men have poorer outcome, regardless of how outcome is defined
Sex-specific differences	Hormonal fluctuations can affect symptom severity	

Ethnicity and race

It was believed in the USA that there were greater rates of schizophrenia in black persons than white persons. A large epidemiological study (the Epidemiologic Catchment Area study in the USA) did not find significant differences between the two groups. It has been thought that schizophrenia has roughly the same prevalence across the world, though this is increasingly debatable. For example, the rates of schizophrenia in Afro-Caribbean immigrants in the UK appear to be significantly higher, perhaps accounted for by the stress of emigration. There also are geographical 'pockets' of higher prevalence rates, as in Northern Sweden and Finland, and Western Ireland. See additional discussion in Chapter 19.

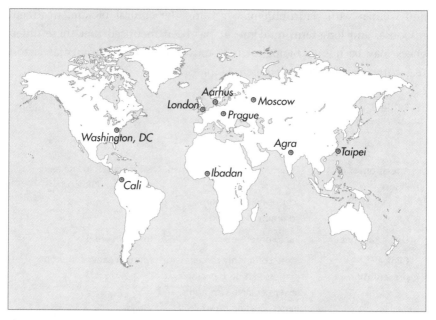

Figure 3.1 Centers where the International Pilot Study of Schizophrenia was conducted.

Culture

Culture (Latin *colere*, to inhabit, to cultivate) defines who we are as individuals. It colors our perceptions, relations with our environment, and notions about health and illness.

CULTURE
- Meanings, values and behavioral norms that are learned and transmitted in the dominant society and within its social groups
- Powerfully influences thinking, feelings and self-concept
- Defines normality and deviance
- Facilitates healthy adaptations
- Has mechanisms that facilitate conflict resolution
- Induces psychopathology by presenting stressors
- Reduces psychopathology by in-built protective factors
- Affects onset, course and outcome of illness
- Shapes tolerance for certain behaviors and clinical symptoms
- Shapes culture-specific expressions of distress

As you can see from the box, culture *is* the human condition. Since cultures vary, individuals originating in those cultures will necessarily have different outlooks. It turns out that there are as many, if not more, differences *within* cultures than across cultures.

> THE CLINICIAN'S CULTURAL COMPETENCY To offer our patients a sense of being understood we must at a minimum be constantly vigilant of how our own cultural perceptions and expectations color every aspect of our clinical interaction. In addition, we need to be culturally aware. This doesn't mean becoming an expert on every culture you are likely to encounter in your practice. Rather, it means that you are inquisitive about other cultures, accepting of differences and non-judgmental about peoples' need to maintain a cultural identity.

Immigration

Immigrants appear to be at heightened risk for developing schizophrenia. One view is that the increased risk is a consequence of stress associated with migration. The alternative view holds that the presence of mental illness itself promotes migration. The interaction between the migrant and the host country is a continuous process, rather than something that happens simply when borders are crossed. The nature of these stresses depends on whether the migrant is a *gastarbeiter* (guest worker), refugee, student, or migrating for economic reasons. Potential sources of stress include interacting with the new socioeconomic systems, the interactions with the host country's culture and changes in the social network of the migrant.

Questions to assess a migrant's experience are:

When did you come here? How old were you?
What were the reasons for moving?
Did you experience difficulties in getting here?
How big was the difference between your birth place and here?
Did you come here alone or in a group?
What are/were you feeling about the new culture?
Did people here help you adjust?
Did/do you feel accepted here?
What has your life been like before you came here?

Asking such questions can go a long way towards acknowledging migrants' challenges in adapting to their new (temporary or permanent) home, validating the complex set of emotions they experience as a result of migration. Sadly, there is an assumption that if individuals *choose* to migrate they ought not to complain about problems. Unfortunately, some immigrants hold the same view, and consequently suffer needlessly. An additional burden that immigrants with schizophrenia contend with is a 'double loss' – first, a life derailed by schizophrenia, and second, forfeiting the typical dream of success in the new land.

Environment

This is a broadly defined category, but includes factors that interact with each other, such as location (urban or rural, industrialized or developing regions), and socioeconomic status (poverty). We will discuss these factors when the issue of who is at risk for schizophrenia is discussed in Chapter 19.

Summary
- Apart from the illness itself, there are biological, environmental and cultural factors that modify the clinical presentation (and long-term outcome).
- Biological factors include sex, race, age and age of onset of illness.
- Environmental factors include, among others, socioeconomic status, social supports, migration, and co-morbid psychiatric and medical conditions.
- There is cultural diversity among patients. Culture has powerful effects on illness presentation, illness perception, and it affects relations with health providers; attention needs to be paid to cultural issues early in assessment and treatment to maximize care of patients.

ANSWERS

Q3.1   RC is a highly educated individual, but this in itself doesn't seem to have direct bearing on the clinical presentation. Ethnicity is an important consideration, but recent research suggests that ethnicity, with few exceptions, may not be a major risk factor. Immigration is frequently cited as a risk factor for schizophrenia. In the case of RC, inquiry about her mental state prior to arriving in the UK may be more important than assuming that voluntary immigration for educational purposes would necessarily increase stress and thereby precipitate psychosis. In all instances one must be sensitive to cultural factors when assessing patients from non-majority cultural backgrounds. With RC we would want to discover whether there are any culturally-derived issues with regard to male professors. RC was 31 years old, an age consistent with the later age at onset of schizophrenia in females, relative to males.

Q3.2 We would guess that MA is female. The age of onset of psychosis in females, relative to males, is mid-20s to early 30s. The presentation with paranoia and depression with acute onset is more commonly seen in females; males tend to have a more insidious onset with fewer mood symptoms. Females tend to have more complete resolution of symptoms with treatment, and generally with few or no negative symptoms. MA's premorbid history is consistent with being female, which tends to evince a better social functioning prior to the onset of illness. By contrast, premorbidly males have substantially more social and school problems.

chapter 4

Schizophrenia, spirituality and religion

We have not lost faith, but we have transferred it from God to the medical profession. George Bernard Shaw (1856–1950)

Prayer is not an old woman's idle amusement. Properly understood and applied, it is the most potent instrument of action.

Mahatma Gandhi (1868–1948)

Although religious institutions used to provide care for the mentally ill in the past, a distancing between religion and psychiatry has occurred since the days of psychoanalysis. In recent years, however, there has been increasing acknowledgment that religion, faith, and spirituality are important dimensions of quality of life, and psychiatry is once again beginning to pay attention to this aspect of personhood.

Defining religion, faith, and spirituality has never been easy, because these precepts cross many boundaries of human activity. Below are simple, hopefully useful definitions. However, regardless of the formal label that one uses (*I'm Buddhist, I'm Roman Catholic, I'm Muslim,* etc.), it is important to ask the patient or the family what *they* hold to be religious or spiritual.

Religion is the belief in the supernatural, sacred, or divine, and the moral codes, practices, values, and institutions associated with such belief. Or we might say that religion is a belief in spiritual beings. But most understand religion to mean organized religion, for example Buddhism, Christianity, Hinduism, Islam, and Judaism.

Faith refers to relational aspects of religion. Among its many meanings are: loyalty to a religion or religious community or its tenets, commitment to a relationship with God and belief in the existence of God.

Spirituality, often used interchangeably with religion, may or may not include belief in supernatural beings and powers, as in religion, but emphasizes experience at a personal level, as in faith. Spirituality can mean a feeling of connectedness, feeling that life has purpose, and that personal development can occur with these perspectives.

Most individuals have had some sort of religious upbringing. Whether they go on to practice that religion, transform their beliefs, or leave behind religion or faith is entirely a matter of personal development. It is important to find out the patient's religious practices because the superimposition of a psychotic disorder on pre-existing beliefs can lead to a complicated set of interactions which need to be sorted out.

Religion and psychosis

Belief in the supernatural (good or evil) is common among people all over the world, and therefore it is no surprise that religious themes are inserted into psychotic phenomena, as are other elements of culture. Religious themes in the context of psychosis include: belief in personal persecution by the devil or equivalent; special messages from, or direct communication with, God; special tasks assigned by the divine; God's voice; and becoming God or one of the supernatural beings. These presentations, although recounted in many texts and religious traditions, would not be considered the norm by most religious practitioners. On the other hand, in many parts of the world there are traditions that are accepting of all of the above. This, however, does not negate the basic premise that a delusion is a fixed, false belief that is at *odds with the community's cultural and religious beliefs*.

When assessing patients presenting with religious delusions it is important, however, not to attribute these beliefs to psychosis alone, but to ascertain the cultural context (Table 4.1). If one is not familiar with the cultural background of the patient, it is the clinician's responsibility to find out.

Good sources of information include family members, clergy, religious organizations, or academics specializing in religious studies.

It is equally important not to assume that all religious expressions in an individual with schizophrenia are pathological, and mistakenly become the target of treatment! Sometimes a resurgence of faith with the onset of illness can be beneficial. Faith can help allay fears and even bring the patient into the orbit of a church or temple community, widening the social network.

Previously held religious beliefs can also become the focus of delusions or hallucinations. It can become difficult to distinguish pathological from normative beliefs under these circumstances. Generally, pathological religious expressions recede with treatment.

Faith can have protective effects. The risk of suicide is lower in patients who have strong belief in traditions forbidding suicide. Substance abuse is likewise decreased because many religions have clear sanctions against intoxicating substances. Prayer is helpful in coping with all sorts of distress, including hallucinations and delusions.

Table 4.1 Distinguishing normative and pathological religious experiences

	Normative religious beliefs	Pathological religiosity
Phenomenology	Consistent with recognized traditions	May or may not be consistent with traditions
Other indicators of psychiatric disturbance	Absent	Present
Mystical or ecstatic experiences	Persons able to revert to reality	Usually a component of psychotic experience, thus unable to control experience
Insight	Generally persons have insight, and understand that others may not share their views	Lacks insight
Time course	Generally long-lasting	Religious delusions may recede with treatment
Lifestyle	Consistent with personal growth	Not necessarily consistent with personal growth

The problem to be faced is: how to combine loyalty to one's own tradition with reverence for different traditions.

Abraham Joshua Heschel (1907–1972)

Religion and the clinician

A clinician's personal religious beliefs or practices ought to have no impact on the assessment and treatment of patients regardless of their beliefs. Further, the clinician must respect the patient's need for spiritual succor and not proselytize. It is also important not to 'pathologize' every form of religious expression in patients, lest we deny them opportunities for the genuine uplift and comfort that can be derived from religion or spirituality.

In order to be sensitive to patients' concerns about religion or faith, it is not necessary to become an expert on all the existing religions and traditions. It is only necessary that the clinician shows interest in these matters, best demonstrated by the nature of questions they ask (*What kinds of religious belief were you brought up with? What are your thoughts about it now? Do you talk to anyone about your religion?*).

Summary
- Religion, faith, and spirituality are important dimensions of quality of life.
- Psychosis and religious beliefs have complex interactions.
- Religious delusions are common, primarily persecutory and grandiose delusions.
- Ascertain the cultural context when assessing patients with religious delusions.
- Do not assume that all religious expressions are pathological.
- Belief can provide comfort and coping skills, be protective (from suicide, substance abuse), and widen the social network. On the other hand, religious delusions can be harmful by provoking violence and suicide, and induce treatment non-adherence.

chapter 5

Putting together the (clinical) pieces

Diagnosis is a system of more or less accurate guessing in which the end-point achieved is a name. These names applied to disease come to assume the importance of specific entities, whereas they are for the most part no more than insecure and therefore temporary conceptions.

Sir Thomas Lewis (1881–1945)

Steps in diagnosis of schizophrenia

Once sufficient current and past psychiatric and medical history has been gathered and a thorough mental status examination conducted, these pieces of information have to be put together to arrive at a 'working diagnosis.' This is the first step in managing the patient's illness.

It is tempting to assign a diagnosis of schizophrenia, or another diagnosis associated with psychosis, when it appears so patently obvious based on the history and mental status exam. In spite of such certitude, it would be highly prudent to consider other possible explanations (see Figure 5.1). There can be serious consequences if a 'short-cut' is taken in the diagnostic process:

- missing a diagnosis that is managed differently from a primary psychosis;
- assigning a diagnosis, such as schizophrenia, that has significant individual and familial psychological effects;
- treating with medications that have potentially serious side effects, some possibly irreversible.

> A woman, aged 30 years, has been experiencing delusions of persecution and grandeur for 9 months along with decreased need for sleep and mood fluctuations. Recently she has been alternating between abusing cocaine and alcohol. She comes to the clinic because of recent onset auditory hallucinations. She reports that she had an automobile accident 6 months ago while intoxicated, requiring hospitalization.

Q5.1 How would you proceed in order to arrive at a working diagnosis?

Could the psychosis be due to a medical condition?

If one uses elevated body temperature as an analog for psychoses, then it becomes easy to appreciate the multitude of causes for psychosis, because psychosis is one expression of deranged brain function. The causes can be broadly categorized according to Table 5.1.

The DSM-IV (Diagnostic and Statistical Manual of Mental Health – IV edn) diagnosis that is assigned for psychosis associated with a medical condition is called **psychotic disorder due to a general medical condition**.

If a medical condition is suspected, then thorough and expeditious investigation should be pursued. A medical history and examination at the beginning are critical to rule out potential reversible causes of schizophrenia-like symptoms. Laboratory studies vary depending on illness history and physical findings, but all 'first-episode' psychotic patients should probably receive brain imaging. Other laboratory studies include complete blood count, electrolyte levels including calcium, thyroid function tests, and sleep-deprived electroencephalogram. However, some researchers have argued that routine endocrine, electroencephalogram and neuroimaging screening tests may not be cost effective. The choice of assessments should be determined by the probability of detection of abnormalities (especially when there is an atypical presentation of the symptoms), cost, invasiveness, and predicted value. Routine use of expensive invasive investigations should be avoided.

Table 5.1 Differential diagnosis of schizophrenia

Cause type	Most common conditions
Neurological	Epilepsies, particularly temporal lobe epilepsy (TLE)
	Cerebrovascular lesions
	Brain trauma
	Huntington's disease
	Hydrocephalus
Metabolic	Wilson's disease
	Porphyrias
	Hartnup disease
Endocrine	Addison's disease
	Cushing's syndrome
	Hyperthyroidism
	Hypothyroidism
	Hyperparathyroidism
Nutritional	Pellagra (B3 deficiency)
	Pernicious anemia (B12 deficiency)
Infectious	Encephalitis
	Cerebral cysts and abscesses
Immune	Addison's disease
	Rheumatic fever
	Multiple sclerosis (MS)
	Systemic lupus erythematosus (SLE)

Could the psychosis be due to substance abuse?

Since substance abuse (alcohol and illicit drugs) is very common, it needs to be ruled out carefully in every instance of psychosis, even when another obvious explanation for psychosis is available. Substance abuse can precipitate psychosis, cause it, and worsen pre-existing psychosis. Common examples of abused substances are:

- Alcohol
- Anxiolytics (e.g. diazepam)
- Cannabis
- Cocaine
- Hallucinogens (e.g. LSD)
- Hypnotics
- Inhalants
- Opioids
- PCP and ketamine
- Sedatives
- Stimulants

The DSM-IV diagnosis assigned for psychosis associated with substance abuse or dependence is called **substance-induced psychotic disorder.** Additional DSM diagnoses for substance abuse or dependence would also be assigned.

Could this be a mood disorder with psychotic features?

Mood disorders can be associated with psychosis. This is generally established by determining first whether the criteria are met for one of the mood disorders and whether the psychosis is present only in the context of the mood disorder. In the DSM-IV-TR, mood disorders with psychotic features are: **major depressive disorder, severe with psychotic features; bipolar I disorder, severe with psychotic features; bipolar II disorder, severe with psychotic features.**

Likelihood of a primary psychotic disorder

The primary psychotic disorders, other than schizophrenia, are shown in Table 5.2.

If the above clinical pathway has got you this far, it is likely that the condition in question is schizophrenia. However, before proceeding to assign an individual with a diagnosis of schizophrenia, one should review the current DSM and ICT criteria as given in Table 5.3.

Table 5.2 Psychotic disorders

Brief psychotic disorder	Characterized by short-lived psychotic symptoms, typically less than 1 month, and frequently in relation to a significant psychosocial stressor. The term 'reactive psychosis' has been used in the literature to describe such cases
Schizophreniform disorder	Schizophrenia-like symptoms of acute onset, perplexity, or other confusion as part of the clinical picture, relatively intact affect, and short duration
Schizoaffective disorder	According to the DSM-IV, the diagnostic criteria of schizoaffective disorder are: a) the presence of major depressive or manic episode concurrent with meeting the diagnostic criteria for the active phase of schizophrenia; b) psychotic symptoms for at least 2 weeks in the absence of prominent affective symptoms during the same episode of illness; and

c) the mood disorder symptoms must be present for a substantial portion of the overall duration of the active and residual periods of the illness. The schizophrenic and affective symptoms can appear simultaneously or in an alternating manner

Delusional disorder

The presence of non-bizarre delusions, that is, involving situations that are plausible, occurring for at least 1 month. The absence of prominent hallucinations. Patients with delusional disorder do not have marked impairment in functioning and do not manifest obviously odd or bizarre behavior. There are several types of delusional disorder as per DSM-IV, classified on the basis of the content of delusions. These include persecutory, jealous, erotomanic, and somatic as well as mixed types of delusional disorder

Shared psychotic disorder

Also called *folie à deux*, characterized by simultaneous occurrence of psychotic symptoms in two or more individuals. It is a rare psychiatric disorder. There are at least three types of this condition:
Folie imposé, characterized by the psychotic symptoms imposed by an individual who has a primary psychotic disorder (the dominant partner) on a submissive, suggestible, and overly dependent relative who lives closely with the person.
Folie simultanée, characterized by the simultaneous onset of similar psychotic symptoms in two closely related individuals who have a close-knit relationship.
Folie communiquée, in which one dominant individual induces additional delusions in an individual who already has some psychotic symptoms.
Folie induite, in which a patient with psychosis adopts another patient's delusion

Culture-bound psychotic disorder

Psychotic syndromes with unique clinical features have been described in a variety of cultures. While in general, the form of symptoms in such syndromes conforms to one or another DSM-IV diagnostic category, the content of phenomena such as hallucinations, delusions, or unusual behaviors are strongly influenced by culture

Table 5.3 Commonly used criteria for the diagnosis of schizophrenia

DSM-IV-TR

The DSM-IV is published by the American Psychiatric Press, USA. For the diagnosis of schizophrenia, the DSM requires the presence of at least two* of the following symptoms present for at least one month:

Delusions
Hallucinations
Disorganized speech
Disorganized or catatonic behavior
Negative symptoms

Additional criteria include the presence of significant decline in (or failure to achieve adequate functioning in) one or more areas of functioning (work, interpersonal relations, or self-care) for a minimum of 6 months, and the exclusion of schizoaffective disorder and mood disorder with psychotic features. Further, it has to be established that the psychosis is not due to the direct physiological effects of a substance (alcohol, drugs of abuse or medications) or a medical condition.

ICD-10

The ICD was developed by the World Health Organization. It is widely used in the UK. The diagnosis of schizophrenia requires the presence, for at least one month, of one well-defined symptom from the following group:

Thought disturbance (thought echo, insertion, withdrawal, or broadcasting)
Delusions of passivity
Persistent delusions
Auditory hallucinations

   or

Two or more symptoms from the following group if the above are absent or not clear-cut:

Persistent hallucinations in any modality
Disturbance in thought processing (derailment, irrelevant speech, neologisms)
Catatonic behavior
Negative symptoms
Significant and consistent changes in behavior (e.g., loss of interest, social withdrawal)

However, schizophrenia should not be diagnosed
In the presence of extensive depressive or manic symptoms (unless the psychosis preceded the mood symptoms):

In the presence of overt brain disease or states of drug intoxication or withdrawal

---

* Only one of these symptoms is needed if a) delusions are bizarre or b)if hallucinations involve a running commentary or conversatione between 2 or more voices.

Next, we want to assign a subtype using formal criteria (DSM or ICD).

Subtypes of schizophrenia (Table 5.4)

- It is more than academic interest that underlies the assignment of subtypes of schizophrenia. Subtypes serve as convenient means (shorthand) for conveying the predominant features of the illness.
- These are broadly classified as paranoid subtype and non-paranoid subtypes (undifferentiated; disorganized, catatonic), and a separate residual subtype.
- Subtypes offer some guidance to prognostication. Patients meeting criteria for paranoid subtype tend to have better outcome than patients diagnosed with non-paranoid subtypes.

Table 5.4. Key features of subtypes of schizophrenia

DSM-IV	ICD-10
Paranoid One or more delusions are prominent or frequent auditory hallucination	**Paranoid** Prominent hallucinations and delusions; disturbances in affect, volition and speech, and catatonia are relatively minimal
Catatonic Catalepsy or stupor, excessive motor activity, extreme negativism, abnormal movement	**Catatonic** One or more of the following symptoms: stupor, excitement, posturing, negativism, rigidity, waxy flexibility or automatism
Undifferentiated Criteria met for schizophrenia, but not for paranoid, disorganized or catatonic subtypes	**Undifferentiated** Criteria met for schizophrenia, but not for paranoid, hebephrenic, catatonic, residual, simple or post-schizophrenic subtypes
Disorganized Prominent disorganized speech or behavior; flat or inappropriate affect	**Hebephrenic** Prominent affective disturbance; delusions and hallucinations are fragmentary/fleeting; unpredictable behavior; flat, inappropriate or silly affect; disorganized speech
Residual Absence of *prominent* symptoms required to diagnose schizophrenia; presence of 2 or more attenuated symptoms, or negative symptoms	**Residual** Prominent negative symptoms; at least one psychotic episode; at least 1-year period when florid psychotic symptoms are minimal
	Simple Insidious and progressive development of behavioral oddities, inability to meet demands of society and decline in overall performance. Delusions and hallucinations are absent
	Post-schizophrenic depression Prominent depression for at least 2 weeks, following schizophrenic illness within the past 12 months (psychosis still present)

- Patients meeting criteria for the non-paranoid subtypes, such as undifferentiated type, tend to have more cognitive deficits and therefore can benefit from cognitive remediation, rehabilitation, etc.
- Subtypes are not static. Over the course of illness the clinical features can change, leading to reassignment of a subtype. The usual direction of change is from paranoid subtype to a non-paranoid subtype.
- Residual subtype indicates that the prominent psychotic phenomena are absent, but stigmata of illness are still present. Return of prominent psychotic symptoms will require reassignment of the subtype.

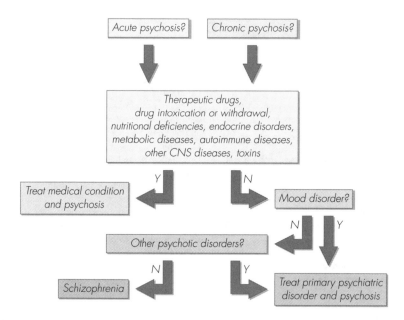

Figure 5.1 Summary of the algorithmic approach to clinical diagnosis of schizophrenia.

ANSWERS

Q5.1 The method (algorithm) shown in Figure 5.1 is the *invariable* process that is utilized to arrive at diagnosis of schizophrenic disorder and assign a subtype. The reasons to exercise care in the diagnostic process are manifold, including missing a diagnosis that is treated differently, labeling an individual with a condition that is stigmatizing, and the emotional trauma that a patient and his or her family will have to endure.

chapter 6

Talking to patients and families

Remember not only to say the right thing in the right place, but far more difficult still, to leave unsaid the wrong thing at the tempting moment.

Benjamin Franklin (1706–1790)

Kind words can be short and easy to speak, but their echoes are truly endless.

Mother Teresa (1910–1997)

The foremost reason for effective communication between clinicians, patients and families is the facilitation and strengthening of the therapeutic alliance (i.e. 'connectedness'), from which stems the best care possible for the patient. The therapeutic bond can help patients and families accept and deal with the illness, improve treatment adherence, and manage crises effectively.

Communication with patients and families often begins on a negative note, commonly when a diagnosis of schizophrenia has been reached and this needs to be conveyed to them. Giving bad news to patients and their families is one of the most onerous tasks for clinicians. Talking to them about schizophrenia is no different, particularly at the time of initial diagnostic assessment. Frequently it is complicated by denial on the part of patient and family.

Reluctance to accept the presence of the illness may be due to:

- fear of stigma
- fear of loss of self-efficacy
- lack of knowledge
- lack of insight
- fear of retaliation by patient or family.

Talking to patients about your assessment

The ability to communicate your findings depends a lot on the severity of the patient's delusions or thought disorder. Patients who are severely ill may not be able to follow your presentation, and a direct approach rarely works, such as

> *I think you have paranoia. We usually see this in schizophrenia . . .*

A better approach might be:

> *You clearly are having difficulties with . . . [symptoms that patient complains about] and I'd like to work with you to help you feel better and also try to figure out what's going on.*
>
> *It seems that you are/were having symptoms such as hearing voices. What you are experiencing appears to be consistent with a condition called psychosis. Many conditions can cause psychosis, including mood disorders and schizophrenia. Have you heard about schizophrenia?*

Talking to patients about treatment

Since antipsychotic drugs are the mainstay of treatment of psychosis, this aspect tends to be emphasized during the early course of the illness. Talking to patients about antipsychotic drugs should be done with the same optimistic stance as one would with any highly treatable condition, particularly at first episode of psychosis. This is because of the very high rates of resolution of the illness with proper treatment.

Patients should be provided with as much detail about their treatment as tolerable to them. If psychosis is interfering with their ability to be a partner in their treatment, then the clinician should continue to engage in a positive therapeutic stance. When the severity of psychosis decreases and the patient becomes more able to discuss treatment, it should be with a long-term view in mind: that treatment is a means to preventing relapses and 'getting back on track'.

> *Call it a clan, call it a network, call it a tribe, call it a family: whatever you call it, whoever you are, you need one.*
>
> Families by Jane Howard (1935–1996)

Talking to families

Generally, the family is the first to notice changes in the patient and may even have been involved in bringing the patient to the hospital or clinic. Nevertheless, the same sensitivity is needed. Families, like patients, are also dealing with the distress of a relative who is acting abnormally (incomprehensibly).

Families respond to a relative's illness in their own unique ways, but typically there are early responses characterized by increased involvement and concern, and with progression of illness a set of late responses, which can include increased criticism. Both sets of responses, if immoderate, can have negative consequences for the patient (Figure 6.1).

All families need reassurance regarding:

- thoroughness of the clinical assessment
- availability of effective treatment
- being informed and consulted about the care of their relative ('kept in the loop')
- that there are others in the same situation ('you're not alone')
- hope.

Statements that don't work:

- *Is anyone in the family schizophrenic? Yes, well that explains it.*
- *Did John have a difficult birth or was he neglected?*

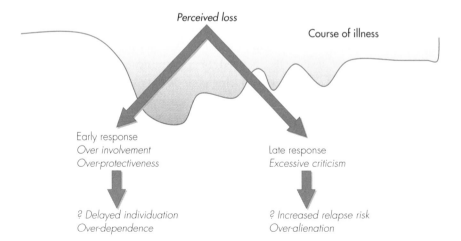

Figure 6.1 Typical family responses to a relative's illness.

Statements that can be helpful:

- *What has it been like for you all with what John's been going through?*
- *What would be helpful to cope with his illness?*

Families often are integral to the care of patients and should be involved from the beginning and offered support. Schizophrenia is an illness that strikes young adults who are likely dependent on their families, and this dependency increases further with illness onset.

What is very helpful is to provide families with the contact telephone numbers of the treatment team, the hospital emergency number, support groups in the neighborhood, and websites with information about schizophrenia.

Family sessions

It is important to meet with families, with and without the patient, as soon as possible after initiating treatment. The goals of family sessions are to allow the sharing of feelings about what is occurring with their relative, provide them with information about the illness, and establish a working alliance with key family members. Involving the family early in the course of treatment can actually help to prevent the patient from alienating him- or herself later. We have found it very useful to insist that initial family sessions include the patient. This largely mitigates any later communication problems between patient and family, between patient and clinician about the family, and between clinician and family. During these sessions we encourage openness, sharing of concerns, talk about the symptoms and the distress, and develop a collaborative spirit (*we'll lick this illness together!*). Also discussed during these sessions is the need for communication between the clinician and the family, particularly during periods of crisis.

When meeting with families, be prepared to answer many, and sometimes difficult, questions. Responses to these questions should be honest, but with a non-judgmental and hopeful stance. The types of information that families seek tend to fall into the following categories:

- definition of psychosis
- triggering factors, role of stress
- substance abuse
- denial, compliance issues
- stigma

- impact of illness on family
- prognosis
- dependence and independence issues
- medications, side effects
- difficulties with healthcare system
- depression, suicide.

NOTE ABOUT CONFIDENTIALITY. Patients have a right to privacy. The therapeutic alliance is fostered when it is clear that confidentiality will be maintained. Family sessions must be approached with this in mind. A general approach is to ask patients whether there is anything they would not like to share with others. Occasionally, patients will forbid outright contact with family. This is a difficult situation, but these wishes must be respected, although every effort must be made to avoid a split between patient and family. We suggest reviewing often the patient's position on this matter because it may alter during treatment. For example, conflicts with family may be due to paranoia, and as it resolves the relations with family improve.

Summary

- Effective communication between clinicians, patients and families facilitates therapeutic alliance, which is essential to good care.
- Talk to patients about treatment with an optimistic stance, particularly since the first episode of psychosis has very high rates of resolution.
- Patients should be provided with as much detail about their treatment as tolerable to them.
- Families, like patients, are also dealing with the stress and trauma of the illness. They also need reassurance that the best is being done for their relative.
- Meet with families as soon as possible, and have at least a few sessions with both patient and family together.
- Be mindful of the confidentiality issues involved in sharing information with family.

chapter 7

Prognostication

Roll the dice, twice, thrice
Pray for me, pay the price
Tell me, tell me Wise One
Will I be the only one?

Once a diagnosis of schizophrenia is made, everyone wants to know what the probable outcome will be. This is very important because, in spite of the best treatments currently available, good outcome is a '50–50' proposition. Prognostication is not yet a science, but there is scientific literature that provides some assistance in conveying to patients, families and others who need to know the odds of a particular outcome, and factors that mediate such outcome.

Questions a **patient and family** may ask when confronted with illness are:
What will happen next?
Will it ever go away?
Why me?

Questions a **health provider** should ask when confronted with illness are:
How can I help now?
How can I help them plan for the future?
How to help them cope with the question, 'why me?'

Prognostication is of great practical importance. To the patient, awareness of the outcome will be critical to make informed life choices as well as to be convinced of the importance of long-term treatment and relapse prevention.

This aspect of the clinician's job needs to be given serious thought, since how such information is presented may make all the difference between a hopeful patient and family who adapt to the illness, versus those who may either deny or grieve the loss, to the detriment of the patient.

Prognostication is a process. It is difficult to determine a likely outcome during the first few days and weeks of the illness. As more information becomes available, such as response to treatment, a more considered opinion can be offered about the future. During the early days of the illness, it is important to maintain a hopeful stance with the patient and family.

BD is a 22-year-old recently diagnosed with schizophrenia. His family wants to know what to expect. BD did very well in school until he experimented with mushrooms a few times, after which he rapidly developed hallucinations and paranoia. He has a very supportive family.

What would you say to the family?

Q7.1 What factors are important in determining BD's prognosis?
a) Gender
b) Age
c) Mushroom abuse
d) Performance in school
e) Rapidity of the onset of psychosis

PREDICTion of outcome

This is of importance both in discussing with patients and family members about what to expect down the road, but also in estimating for return to employment that is needed for most occupational disability evaluations. Fortunately, a substantial body of evidence exists to guide the clinician in answering this question at least with some level of confidence. The following factors have been thought to have some predictive value.

Premorbid maladjustment
Resource limitations
Early onset
Delay in treatment
Inadequate treatment
Cognitive impairment
Treatment non-response

Table 7.1 Prognostic factors

Favorable factors	Unfavorable factors
Being female	Being male
Later onset of illness	Early onset of illness
Obvious precipitating factors	Withdrawn, autistic behavior
Acute onset	Insidious onset
Good premorbid social, sexual, and work histories	Neurological signs and symptoms
Mood disorder symptoms (especially depressive)	History of perinatal trauma
Married	No remission in three years
Family history of mood disorders	Family history of schizophrenia
Good support systems	History of assaultiveness
Positive symptoms	Prominent negative symptoms
Good recovery between episodes	Many relapses
	Lower premorbid IQ

A useful way of developing a prognostic evaluation is to sort out for each patient those factors indicative of a favorable prognosis and stack them against factors associated with unfavorable prognosis (Table 7.1). Based on the best available clinical and research information, a thoughtful, realistic, yet hopeful assessment regarding the future should be offered to the patient and family. Such discussions should occur periodically because new information or treatments are always forthcoming.

Another facet of outcome in schizophrenia is the *path* to the long-term outcome. As can be seen in Figure 7.1 there are several pathways that the illness can take during the course of several years. Prediction of a specific illness course early on is difficult to determine.

LK has a 2-year history of schizophrenia. He had a very good treatment response at first episode of illness, enabling return to full-time school. One year later he relapsed, requiring hospitalization. He returned to school but could manage only one course. Recently he relapsed again and now requires a group home.

Q7.2 What is LK's course of illness?
a) Single, unremitting episode
b) Episodic, *without* inter-episode deficits
c) Episodic, *with* inter-episode deficits
d) Chronic, deteriorating

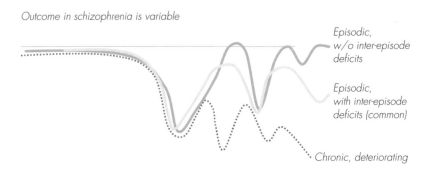

Outcome in schizophrenia is variable

Episodic,
w/o inter-episode
deficits

Episodic,
with inter-episode
deficits (common)

Chronic, deteriorating

Figure 7.1 Illness course

Summary

- Prognostication is very important because, in spite of the best treatments currently available, outcome is somewhat unpredictable.
- Prognostication is critical to making informed life choices, planning long-term management.
- Prognostication is a *process*: as more information becomes available with the passage of time, more thoughtful opinion regarding the future can be offered.
- During the early days of the illness, it is important to maintain a hopeful stance with the patient and family.
- There are a variety of patient-related and treatment-related factors that are helpful in prognostication.

ANSWERS

Q7.1 Being male is generally a risk factor for poorer long-term outcome. BD's onset of illness is at the upper age range for males (late adolescence to early adulthood), which is more favorable than later age at onset. Drug abuse is commonly observed before and during onset of illness, and may not specifically be prognostic unless it becomes chronic. Good premorbid school functioning favors a better outcome. Likewise, rapid onset of illness is associated with good outcome. In summary, although BD is male with a usual age at onset of illness, he has several factors in favor of a likely good outcome. Further, he has a supportive family which also bodes well for BD.

Q7.2 LK is showing evidence for a chronic, deteriorating course. On the other hand, if LK's course of illness had been examined one year ago, it might have appeared to be episodic, with inter-episode deficits. Thus, the course of illness is determined retrospectively.

chapter 8

Phase-specific treatment

Little by little does the trick.   Aesop (6th century BC)

The aim of treatment is full and lasting **recovery**, a notion that includes the complete absence of symptoms and return to premorbid level of functioning. Some definitions of recovery also include no further requirement for treatment and no longer being viewed as psychiatrically ill. Recovery, as defined by these stringent criteria, occurs in relatively few patients with schizophrenia. However, many patients can achieve satisfactory levels of treatment response that significantly improves the quality of life.

The first steps towards recovery are to achieve maximal symptom control and psychosocial functioning and minimize the burden of treatment. This is accomplished by combining pharmacological and psychosocial modalities, followed by rehabilitation.

Since schizophrenia is a life-long disorder, treatment should be tailored to the specific phases of the illness course – psychotic phase, convalescence, and stable phase (Figure 8.1). The advantages of phase-specific treatment are the multidimensional approach to managing the illness and its consequences and comprehensive planning for this life-long illness (Table 8.1).

Each phase has specific treatment issues – pharmacotherapy ('brain-focused' treatment) and psychotherapy ('person-focused' treatment) (Table 8.2). As treatment progresses additional social and rehabilitative services likely will be required. Treatment phases do not progress in neat linear fashion: the transition from one phase to the next tends to be fuzzy.

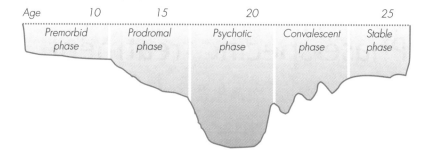

Figure 8.1 Natural course of schizophrenia depicting the critical phases of the illness.

Table 8.1 The 'Six Rs' of phase-specific treatment

Phase	Treatment goals
Psychotic	**R**ecognition of psychosis
	Response to the psychosis – treatment
Convalescent	**R**emission of most disturbing symptoms
	Relapse prevention by promoting treatment adherence
Stable	**R**eintegrate into the community; reduce secondary morbidity
	Rehabilitation

Table 8.2 Overview of phase-specific treatment issues

Psychotic phase	Convalescence	Stable phase
Agitation & insomnia	**Co-morbid**	**Monitoring treatment**
Short acting	**depression, anxiety**	Monitoring compliance
benzodiazepines	Adjunct antidepressants/	Relapse prevention
IM olanzapine or	mood stabilizers/	
ziprasidone	anxiolytics	
Psychotic symptoms	**Treatment**	
Selection and titration	**resistance**	
of an atypical	Clozapine	
antipsychotic drug		

Acute side effects
Dose adjustment
Achieve minimal
effective dose
Adjunct
anticholinergic/ beta
blockers

Non-compliance
Maintenance
treatments
Depot medications

**Denial, fear,
treatment refusal**
Establishment of
therapeutic alliance

**Post-psychotic
depression**
Suicidality
Supportive/cognitive
psychotherapy
Increased vigilance
Support

**Developmental
issues**
Interactions in
groups with other
young people at
similar illness
stage

Agitation, psychosis
Removal from
stressful environment
Reduce stimulation
Cognitive behavioral therapy

**Continuing
delusions**
Engage in cognitive
therapy

**Deficits in social
cognition**
Cognitive remediation
Social skills training

Lack of knowledge
Education focused on
symptoms/syndromes
(psychosis)
Involve family

Substance misuse
Substance abuse
groups

Stress
Hypercritical/uninvolved
family stigma
Educate family
Teach patient coping
and stress
management skills
Public education

Non-compliance
Continued illness
education
Maintain therapeutic
alliance

**Dependence/
independence issues**
Gradual, stepwise
move to independence
Vocational
rehabilitation

General principles of treatment

At the outset

The chances of a favorable outcome are improved if the following are established at the outset:

- Therapeutic alliance
- Collaboration
- Education

Therapeutic alliance is the working relationship between patient and clinician that facilitates all activities required for treatment. Research has shown that therapeutic alliance is very important to good treatment outcome. Even if patients are floridly psychotic the therapeutic stance should be always maintained.

Collaboration is a component of therapeutic alliance, but more specifically it is the tacit understanding between patient and clinician that treatment will be undertaken jointly. Rather than being a passive recipient of treatment, the patient, to the extent that she or he can, will be a partner in the process. The clinician, rather than 'handing out' treatment will take a collaborative stance and solicit feedback from the patient. A successful collaboration is when it is 'we' who will battle the illness rather than 'you' or 'me'.

Education about the illness and its treatment are very important for both patient and his or her family. Psychoeducation facilitates treatment compliance, recognition of signs of relapse, managing side effects and persistent symptoms. Psychoeducation is a process that continues throughout the different phases of treatment, may require modification according to the patient's clinical condition, and repeated often.

The next steps

- Consenting process
- Medical clearance
- Identify target symptoms
- Plan the duration of medication trial
- Anticipate and monitor side effects
- Monitor compliance
- Plan *'Plan B'*

Consenting process is both a legal requirement and a therapeutic necessity. Patients have a right to know the nature of the treatment. It is a *process* because the ability to consent in full measure depends on the severity of cognitive deficits. The presence of psychosis *per se* doesn't interfere with the consenting process. Further, in the spirit of collaboration, majority of patients and their families appreciate being informed about the specifics of treatment.

Medical clearance may be required before initiating treatment if there are concerns about medical co-morbidity or to establish a baseline before initiating treatment.

Identify target symptoms in order to track the effectiveness of treatment. Different symptoms will resolve at different rates. Vegetative symptoms (sleep and appetite disturbance) tend to show the earliest change, and positive symptoms improve before negative symptoms. Keeping your eye on a key set of symptoms provides a useful means of gauging treatment response. We have recently begun using the Simplified Clinical Assessment of Psychosis (SCAP), described in Figure 8.2, to follow treatment progress.

Plan the duration of medication trial even though it is not possible to predict treatment response. Most treatment trials at adequate dose are 8–12 weeks long. The advantage of planning a treatment trial is to alert the patient that some amount of patience is required. On the other hand, if a medication is having no effect at all, then changing treatment earlier than the planned duration is prudent. The longer the psychosis remains unabated the greater the risk for chronicity.

Anticipate and monitor side effects in order to deal with them early and effectively (Chapters 9 and 12). Addressing side effects early reduces the risk of treatment non-adherence. It is best to inquire about side effects at each visit. Some patients are not forthcoming about side effects, particularly sexual dysfunction, and require direct questioning.

Monitor compliance because treatment non-adherence is a very common problem (Chapter 14).

Plan to have alternative treatments in mind (*Plan B*), whether you utilize a standardized treatment algorithm or your own practice methods, because it offers hope to patients. It is very relieving for patients and families to know that there are many treatment options in the event that the current regimen fails.

NAME or ID: _____ TIME POINT: _____ RATER: _____DATE: _____

1. **DELUSIONS**   ☐
    1. No delusional thinking
    2. Overvalued ideas
    3. Delusions (including paranoia) – do not significantly impair functioning
    4. Delusions – interfere with functioning but allow engagement in the interview
    5. Delusions that prevent engagement during the interview

2. **HALLUCINATIONS**   ☐
    1. No hallucinations
    2. Illusions or hallucinations that occur infrequently
    3. Frequent hallucinations that do not significantly impair functioning
    4. Hallucinations – interfere with functioning but allow engagement during the interview
    5. Hallucinations that prevent engagement during the interview

3. **THOUGHT DISORDER**   ☐
    1. Linear thinking
    2. Circumstantial thinking or occasional tangentiality
    3. Tangential thinking or occasional derailment
    4. Derailment and/or thought blocking
    5. Largely incomprehensible speech

4. **ALOGIA**   ☐
    1. Adequate and spontaneous speech production
    2. Brief answers; little spontaneity; questions are required to move interview along
    3. Very brief or monosyllabic responses; directed questions are required for moving interview along
    4. Few questions answered
    5. Mutism

5. **AFFECT**   ☐
    1. Normal affect
    2. Mildly restricted affect
    3. Restricted affect and/or inappropriate affect
    4. Blunted affect
    5. Flat affect

TOTAL SCORE OF ABOVE ITEMS   ☐

GLOBAL ASSSESSMENT OF PSYCHOSIS (GAP)   ☐
    1. No psychosis
    2. Mild psychosis
    3. Moderate psychosis
    4. Moderately severe psychosis
    5. Severe psychosis

Figure 8.2 Simplified clinical assessment of psychosis (SCAP).

Summary
- The aim of treatment is full and lasting recovery.
- The first steps towards recovery are maximal symptom control and psychosocial functioning and minimizing the burden of treatment, utilizing pharmacotherapy, psychosocial therapies, and rehabilitation.
- Phase-specific treatment utilizes multidimensional approaches to managing the illness during the psychotic phase, convalescence and stable phase.
- Treatment phases do not progress neatly and the transition from one phase to the next tends to be fuzzy.
- Each phase has specific treatment issues – pharmacotherapy ('brain-focused' treatment) and psychotherapy ('person-focused' treatment).
- The chances of a favorable outcome are improved if the following are established at the outset: **therapeutic alliance, collaboration, and education.**
- The next steps in initiating treatment are to obtain consent, medical clearance, identify target symptoms, have an idea of the duration of the treatment trial, anticipate and monitor side effects, monitor compliance, and plan for alternative treatments in the event of current trial fails.

chapter 9

Managing symptoms: pharmacological approach

The patient does not care about your science; what he wants to know is, can you cure him?   Martin H. Fischer (1879–1962)

The treatment of schizophrenia was revolutionized in 1952 with the use of chlorpromazine as the first effective pharmacological antipsychotic. In the intervening half century numerous antipsychotic agents have come to market. This latter fact is important because it offers several options in the event that the first, second or more antipsychotic agents do not yield an optimal treatment response.

What are antipsychotic agents?

These are a diverse group of drugs that are used to treat psychotic symptoms. These drugs are not specifically antischizophrenia, but are used to treat any condition associated with psychosis. Antipsychotic drugs (APDs) used to be referred to as major tranquilizers (inducing calm) or neuroleptics (*lepsis*, to hold down).

During the first 30 years since chlorpromazine, attention was focused on drugs that blocked the neurotransmitter dopamine. In the intervening years, research shifted to other neurotransmitters, particularly serotonin. Since the late 1980s, the so-called 'second generation' APDs have emerged as front-runners in the treatment of schizophrenia. The 'first generation' APDs are also referred to as *typical* neuroleptics, indicating that they are primarily dopamine-blocking drugs, and the newer APDs are referred to as *atypical* APDs because they have different mechanisms of action, affecting in most

Table 9.1 Advantages and disadvantages of APDs

	Advantages	*Disadvantages*
Typical APDs (e.g. haloperidol, fluphenazine, thiothixene)	• Effective with positive symptoms • Low risk of metabolic syndrome • Haloperidol useful in delirium, pregnancy	• No effect on negative symptoms • No effect on cognitive deficits • Extrapyramidal syndromes (EPS) • Prolactin elevation
Atypical APDs (e.g. aripiprazole, clozapine, olanzapine, quetiapine, risperidone, ziprasidone)	• Effective with positive and negative symptoms, and cognitive deficits • Low EPS potential[1] • Little prolactin elevation[2]	• Weight gain[3] • Increased risk of metabolic syndrome • Expensive

1. Risperidone at higher doses induces EPS with greater frequency.
2. Risperidone tends to increase prolactin levels.
3. Greatest weight gain is seen with clozapine and olanzapine.

cases both dopamine and serotonin neurotransmission. You will discover, however, that *typical* and *atypical* labeling reflects convenience (which is why we will use it throughout the book) rather than scientific labelling.

All APDs have variable degrees of advantages and disadvantages, the salience of which depends on the clinical situation at hand (see Table 9.1).

Starting antipsychotic treatment

Before prescribing treatment, become familiar with all the atypical APDs (there are not that many!), clozapine in particular, as well as a few typical APDs, particularly the high-potency agents (e.g. haloperidol, fluphenazine).

The two most common clinical situations that require initiation of APDs are (i) first-episode psychosis and (ii) relapse following discontinuation of treatment by the patient. Switching APDs can occur at any time during the course of illness, whether it is due to intolerable side effects or suboptimal treatment response.

Initiation of APDs for **first-episode psychosis** requires consideration of the clinical presentation, the treatment setting and concerns about specific side effects. Risperidone, olanzapine, quetiapine, ziprasidone or aripiprazole are equally effective. There is no clear data that can help choose among these drugs based on efficacy. In general, the choice depends on what side effects one wishes to *avoid* in a given patient. Patients at first-episode of psychosis are prone to side effects. Therefore, the starting dose should be low, dose increases should be in small increments, and side effects should be addressed quickly, lest the patient become treatment non-adherent. Patients at first-episode of psychosis tend to have very good treatment response. The research evidence and our own studies indicate quite good treatment response (>70%).

Initiation of APDs following **discontinuation of treatment** by the patient requires ascertaining previous treatment history. In general, an APD that has worked well in the past is likely to be a good first choice. When such information is not available, the choice may be made based on what side effects one wishes to avoid.

Current standards of practice increasingly favor atypical APDs as first-line treatment, although typical APDs still have important roles in the treatment of schizophrenia, particularly in first-episode patients. The brief descriptions of common atypical APDs in Table 9.2 is to familiarize you with their usage characteristics; it is *not* all the information you need for their use in specific patients. You will need to refer to pharmacopeias for details about pharmacodynamics, metabolism and side effects of these drugs.

Drug selection

As noted earlier, there is no convincing research data that can help in choosing one APD over another based on efficacy alone, particularly among the atypical APDs. One approach is to choose an APD based on side effects one wishes to *avoid* (Table 9.3), along with other considerations such as previous treatment response, preference, route and frequency of administration, and cost.

Table 9.2 Prescriptive characteristics of some common atypical APDs.

Olanzapine

Trade names	**Zyprexa, Zydis**
Available dosing (mg)	2.5, 5, 7.5, 10, 15, 20; Zydis 5, 10, 15, 20
Starting dose	5–10 mg daily
Usual daily dose	5–20 mg
Maximum daily dose	40 mg
Elderly dosing	Start at 2.5–5 mg; 3–15 mg daily
Child dosing	5–10 mg daily
Adolescent dosing	10–15 mg daily
Metabolism	CYP450: 1A2; 2D6

Risperidone

Trade names	**Risperdal, Risperdal Consta**
Available dosing (mg)	0.25, 0.5, 1, 2, 4, 1/ml solution; Consta IM
Starting dose	1–2 mg daily
Usual daily dose	1–4 mg daily
Maximum daily dose	16 mg
Elderly dosing	Starting 0.25–0.5 mg daily; 0.5–4 mg daily
Child dosing	1–2 mg daily
Adolescent dosing	2.5–4 mg daily
Metabolism	CYP450: **2D6**; 3A4

Quetiapine

Trade name	**Seroquel**
Available dosing (mg)	25, 100, 200, 300
Starting dose	100 mg daily
Usual daily dose	400–600 mg
Maximum daily dose	800 mg
Elderly dosing	50–300 mg daily
Child dosing	150–400 mg daily
Adolescent dosing	250–550 mg daily
Metabolism	CYP450: 2D6; **3A4**

Ziprasidone

Trade name	**Geodon**
Available dosing (mg)	20, 40, 60, 80
Starting dose	20–40 mg daily
Usual daily dose	40 mg
Maximum daily dose	80 mg
Elderly dosing	20–80 mg daily
Child dosing	40–100 mg daily
Adolescent dosing	80–140 mg daily
Metabolism	CYP450: **3A4**

Aripiprazole

Trade name	**Abilify**
Available dosing (mg)	5, 10, 15, 20, 30
Starting dose	10–15 mg daily
Usual daily dose	10–15 mg
Maximum daily dose	30 mg
Elderly dosing	10–25 mg daily
Child dosing	10–15 mg daily
Adolescent dosing	250–550 mg daily
Metabolism	CYP450: 2D6, **3A4**; poor 2D6 metabolizers have 60% increased drug exposure

Clozapine

Trade name	**Clozapine**
Available dosing (mg)	12.5, 25, 100
Baseline testing?	White blood count (WBC), repeated weekly for 6 months, then biweekly
Starting dose	12.5–25 mg daily
Usual daily dose	300–600 mg
Maximum daily dose	900 mg
Elderly dosing	100–400 mg daily
Child dosing	100–350 mg daily
Adolescent dosing	225–450 mg daily
Metabolism	CYP450: **1A2**; 2D6; **3A4**

Table 9.3 Selection of APD based on side-effect profile

Side effect being avoided	Preferred APD
Sedation and weight gain	Risperidone, ziprasidone, high potency conventional antipsychotic
Extrapyramidal syndromes	Clozapine, quetiapine, olanzapine, ziprasidone, risperidone, low potency conventional antipsychotic
Cognitive side effects	Atypical antipsychotics
Anticholinergic side effects	Risperidone, ziprasidone, quetiapine
Reproductive side effects	Quetiapine, olanzapine, ziprasidone, clozapine
Cardiovascular side effects	Risperidone, olanzapine, quetiapine, high potency neuroleptic

Drug titration and treatment duration

When initiating treatment, almost always *start low, go slow*. The aim of treatment is to arrive at maximal therapeutic benefit using the lowest effective dose while minimizing side effects. This is best achieved with the 'low and slow' approach. Decreasing the likelihood of side effects will enhance treatment adherence, in turn improving treatment response.

Most patients respond to 300–700 mg chlorpromazine *equivalents* (relative potency of APDs compared to a standard dose of chlorpromazine). Table 9.4 provides chlorpromazine equivalents of common APDs.

The issue of duration of treatment in reality reflects the following:

- *How long to continue the APD at the dose effective for the acute phase?*
- *How long is treatment continued when symptoms have remitted?*
- *How long is an adequate treatment trial?*
- *Can treatment ever be stopped?*

Patients and families tend to be concerned mostly about the last question. Evidence suggests the treatment in most instances needs to be continued for life. After remission of an acute episode the same APD and the dose that was effective should be maintained for at least a year and probably longer. Discontinuing treatment at any point increases the risk of relapse. There are rare patients who have one episode of psychosis that remits completely; in such patients discontinuing APDs may be considered. In all other patients with schizophrenia, treatment should be viewed as lifelong.

Table 9.4 Chlorpromazine equivalents

Chlorpromazine	100 mg
Haloperidol	2 mg
Fluphenazine	2 mg
Risperidone	2 mg
Olanzapine	5 mg
Quetiapine	75 mg
Ziprasidone	60 mg
Aripiprazole	7.5 mg
Haloperidol decanoate	5 mg every 4 weeks
Fluphenazine decanoate	10 mg every 2 weeks

Common problems during a psychotic episode

Arousal and agitation

There can be many reasons for an agitated state. Patients with paranoia are fearful and may become aggressive as a means of self-defense. Agitation can also be due to irritability, intoxication, substance abuse and withdrawal states, and akathisia (drug-induced restlessness), all of which can be present alongside schizophrenia. The first order of business is safety of patient and staff. This may include seclusion and restraints, but only as a last resort. There has been a move away from using APDs as first-line treatment of agitation, although they are still used in certain situations (see Chapter 16). Short-term benzodiazepines, such as lorazepam or clonazepam, have been found to be very effective in decreasing agitation with relatively few undesirable side effects. An advantage of benzodiazepines is their availability in both oral and parenteral formulations (see Appendix B). It is preferable to offer oral preparations before resorting to intramuscular (IM) injections. In the event that benzodiazepines are ineffective, APDs can be used. IM olanzapine or ziprasidone are newer preparations that can be used in managing arousal that is non-responsive to other measures (see Appendix B). APDs are associated with significantly more side effects requiring vigilance.

Insomnia

The quantity of sleep, its initiation and maintenance are frequently affected in schizophrenia, particularly during florid states. Lack of adequate sleep can contribute to irritability and exacerbation of psychosis. Some APDs have sedation as an early side effect that can be advantageous in this situation. If insomnia persists, short-term oral benzodiazepines can be utilized (e.g. temazepam 10–20 mg, clonazepam 1–2 mg), or a hypnotic, (e.g. zopiclone 7.5 mg or zolpidem 5–10 mg). These drugs should be used sparingly, because of their addictive potential. Chronic insomnia requires systematic evaluation and management. Referral to a sleep evaluation clinic is appropriate.

Summary

- APDs are a diverse group of drugs used to treat psychotic symptoms, not just schizophrenia.
- Typical APDs are referred to as 'first generation' neuroleptics, and are primarily dopamine-blocking drugs. Atypical, or 'second generation', APDs

have different mechanism of action, affecting dopamine and serotonin neurotransmission.

- There are no clear data that can help choose among APDs based on efficacy alone. One approach is to choose an APD based on the side effects one wants to avoid.
- When an APD is being restarted choose an APD that has worked well in the past.
- Atypical APDs are increasingly used as first-line treatment for first-episode patients with schizophrenia.
- ***Start low, go slow*** when initiating treatment.
- Most patients respond to 300–700 mg chlorpromazine equivalents.
- Maintain the effective APD dose at least for a year.
- Treatment is likely to be lifelong for most patients with schizophrenia.

chapter 10

Managing symptoms: psychosocial approaches

You gain strength, courage, and confidence by every experience in which you really stop to look fear in the face. You are able to say to yourself, 'I have lived through this horror. I can take the next thing that comes along.'

Eleanor Roosevelt (1884–1962)

While antipsychotic drugs (APDs) are largely effective in controlling the severity of positive symptoms, many patients continue to experience distressing delusions and hallucinations. Even with the newer APDs, improvements in overall disability are limited. Thus, a comprehensive approach to overall management is critically important, which includes individual, group, and community-based psychosocial treatments. It is easy to forget – because of the initial focus on the pharmacotherapy of positive symptoms – that psychosocial treatments are integral to treating schizophrenia from the outset, not as an afterthought. Just as there have been many advances in pharmacotherapy, there have been recent major advances in a variety of psychosocial treatment modalities.

The main forms of psychosocial interventions are:

- Psychoeducation
- Cognitive behavioral therapy
- Compliance therapy
- Cognitive remediation.

Psychoeducation

A succession of eye-openers each involving the repudiation of some previously held belief.   George Bernard Shaw (1856–1950)

Psychoeducational approaches increase patients' knowledge of, and insight into, their illness and its treatment, enabling people with schizophrenia to cope with their illness in more effective ways, thereby improving prognosis. Several clinical trials have shown that psychoeducation programs reduce relapse, improve symptomatic recovery, and enhance psychosocial and family outcomes. To be successful, psychoeducation needs to be timely, repeated as necessary, and tailored to the patient or family members' cultural and educational background. Individual and group settings, as well as family groups, are effective.

While there are many variations of psychoeducation, they all embrace a set of core principles that are aimed at maximizing the chances of recovery through education. Our version of psychoeducation has two components (Table 10.1): **TEACH**, which focuses on the process of conveying information; and **I'M SCARED**, which describes the content of the education that addresses the fears that patients and families have about how to cope with the illness and what the future holds for them. The key elements of the program are listed in Table 10.1.

Table 10.1 Psychoeducation principles

TEACH	I'M SCARED
Timely: provide education early	**I**nternal monitoring of mental state & meaning of psychosis
Empower: give as much control as possible to patient/family	**M**edication effects – positive & negative effects
Adapt education to match educational, cultural background	**S**tigma
Continuous education: repeat often; confirm understanding	**C**oping skills to reduce stress
Hopeful: positive; avoid premature labeling/ prognostication	**A**llying with family, friends and clinicians
	Relapse recognition
	Evolving – planning for the future
	Drug abuse prevention

Cognitive behavioral therapy (CBT)

Men are disturbed not by things, but by the view which they take of them.

Epictetus (55–135 AD)

Cognitive behavioral therapy (CBT), aims to realign negative or distorted thinking in order to reduce distress. It has been an evolving treatment modality since the 1950s and has been extensively applied in the treatment of depression, anxiety disorders and personality disorders.

Cognitive behavioral therapy focuses on identifying situations and thoughts that are associated with distress, finding acceptable alternative perspectives and then practicing new ways of thinking and behaving outside the therapy session (i.e. homework). Because CBT requires patients to have the capability of participating actively in these methods, there has been reluctance to utilizing it for schizophrenia, because psychosis was presumed to interfere with the conduct of CBT. Fortunately, CBT has been found to be useful for patients with schizophrenia. It is effective in reducing persistent positive symptoms in chronic patients and may even speed recovery in acutely ill patients. There is much research ongoing to determine whether CBT reduces relapse rates.

In CBT, symptoms such as delusions and hallucinations are seen as stemming from information-processing biases such as the tendency to overestimate coincidences, jump to conclusions, attribute internal events to external sources, and blame others when things are not going well.

SOME TERMS USED IN CBT

- **Automatic thoughts** come to mind when a particular situation occurs leading to maladaptive behavior. CBT aims to challenge automatic thoughts.
- **Cognitive restructuring** is the process of replacing maladaptive (negative) thought patterns (schemas) with constructive and positive thoughts and beliefs.
- **Relaxation techniques** used to relieve stress, include biofeedback, meditation and exercise.
- **Schemas** are core beliefs or assumptions that serve as filters through which we view the world.

Compliance therapy

There is some evidence that a new therapeutic technique known as compliance therapy (CT) can help to improve treatment adherence in schizophrenia. Treatment non-adherence is a major concern in the management of schizophrenia (see Chapter 14).

Compliance therapy is based on brief motivational interviewing and cognitive therapy techniques. CT has shown to result in greater improvements in the patients' attitudes to drug treatment, insight and treatment adherence, as well as a trend for lower hospital admission rates. Typically, CT involves 4–6 sessions of 20–60 minutes each.

The ABCs of CT

- *Assessment and alliance building.* Review the patient's history; formulate patient's approach to treatment; link medication discontinuation and relapse (ask the patient: *Do you think there is a link between you stopping the medicine and ending back in the hospital?*).
- *Behavior change.* Explore the ambivalence towards treatment; help patient identify benefits and disadvantages.
- *Consolidation.* Encouraging self-efficacy; reframing medication as a way to enhance quality of life.

Cognitive remediation

Cognitive dysfunction, now considered a fundamental feature of schizophrenia affecting 40–95% of individuals, contributes significantly to disability.

Cognitive functions affected in schizophrenia are:

- attention
- working memory (e.g. capacity to keep things in mind long enough for immediate use, such as a phone number)
- learning
- general memory
- forward planning
- concept formation
- initiating action
- self-monitoring.

Cognitive remediation involves repeated practice and the learning strategies that enhance compensatory strategies to 'bypass' some of the cognitive deficits. Cognitive remediation strategies vary widely in duration, intensity, method, target of behavioral intervention, and clinical status of participants. Using these approaches, improvements have been observed on measures of working memory, emotion perception, and executive function. One form of cognitive remediation called cognitive enhancement therapy (CET), developed by researchers at Pittsburgh, focuses on deficits related to social cognition (the ability to act wisely in social interactions) thought to impede social and vocational recovery. Social cognition is acquired during adolescence and early adulthood. CET is designed to facilitate the individual's transition from prepubertal to young-adult style of social cognition. The treatment involves helping the individual to develop a 'gistful' appraisal of interpersonal behavior and novel social contexts.

Managing specific symptoms

In spite of optimal treatment, about a third of patients experience persistent hallucinations and delusions which can be quite distressing. A variety of strategies can be offered to help patients cope and even reduce the severity of hallucinations (Table 10.2) and delusions (Table 10.3).

Table 10.2 ABCs of coping with hallucinations

Arousal reduction	Relaxation and deep breathing exercises
	Blocking ears, closing eyes
	Listening to music
Behavior	Increasing non-social activity
	Reality testing
	Seeking opinions from others
Cognition	Distraction
	Ignoring
	Positive self-talk

Table 10.3 Delusions **BARRED**

Become aware	Increase awareness of delusional thoughts and assumptions
Alternative explanations	Utilize alternative (more neutral) explanations for delusional thought
Record Relaxation techniques	Monitor and record delusional thoughts Deep breathing and distraction techniques
Esteem	Improving self-esteem helps cope with delusions of low worth (often due to derogatory auditory hallucinations)
Double book keeping	A mental trick of being able to keep two incongruent ideas in mind without undue distress. For example, believing that one is a millionaire yet living within very limited means

Summary

- While APDs are very effective for psychosis, psychosocial treatments are critically important to reduce overall disability.
- The main forms of psychosocial interventions are: **psychoeducation, cognitive behavioral therapy, compliance therapy,** and **cognitive remediation**.
- Psychoeducational approaches increase patients' knowledge of, and insight into, their illness and its treatment.
- Cognitive behavioral therapy (CBT) focuses on identifying situations and thoughts that are associated with distress, finding acceptable alternative perspectives, and then practicing new ways of thinking and behaving outside the therapy session.
- Compliance therapy (CT) can help to improve treatment adherence in schizophrenia.
- Cognitive remediation involves learning strategies that enhance compensatory strategies to 'bypass' some of the cognitive deficits common in schizophrenia.
- A third of patients experience persistent hallucinations and delusions which can be improved by utilizing a combination of the above techniques.

chapter 11

Rehabilitation: road to recovery

The rung of a ladder was never meant to rest upon, but only to hold a man's foot long enough to enable him to put the other somewhat higher.

Thomas Henry Huxley (1825–1895)

Rehabilitation (from Latin *habilitas*, to make able) has many meanings, but common to these definitions is the notion of returning to the highest possible level of functioning, whether it is physical, psychological, social, or environmental. The definition implies a loss of functioning from a previous higher level due to disease or disuse.

Rehabilitation is critical to recovery because pharmacological and psychosocial treatments are not very effective means to recovering the previous level of functioning. Pharmacological and psychosocial treatments can be viewed as bringing the patient to the threshold of recovery by symptom remission, while rehabilitation is the process by which the threshold is crossed, leading to recovery and improved quality of life.

Rehabilitation is not a single technique or method; rather it is a collection of activities that address a multiplicity of needs which patients with schizophrenia encounter even after symptom control. Rehabilitation can be thought of as achieving **HOPE** for patients through the following:

Housing
Occupation
People and networks
Economic independence

Rehabilitation methods

Case management

Treat people as if they were what they ought to be, and you help them to become what they are capable of being.

Goethe (1749–1832)

Case management is about helping patients negotiate their environment so as to maximize recovery. Treatment of schizophrenia can be a confusing choreography, involving visits to the doctor for follow-up care, obtaining medications, attending groups and rehabilitation activities, arranging transportation for these visits, and so forth. Attending to these tasks can be a challenge for patients, even during the recovering phase. Faltering by the patient in attending to different aspects of treatment can increase the risk of relapse. Case management, which includes a wide range of activities such as outreach, crisis intervention, public education, and resource management, can be highly effective in maintaining patients in the community and in improving outcome. Intensive case management, also termed assertive community treatment, has been found to reduce hospital admission rates and family burden.

Intensive case management (ICM), a variation of case management, serves as a liaison between inpatient and outpatient care, including discharge planning and links to community programs.

Assertive community treatment

Assertive community treatment (ACT) offers a continuity of medical, psychiatric, and social services to patients in the community utilizing mobile outreach clinical teams with the aim of keeping patients out of the hospital. A combination of services is used, such as case management, social service entitlements, housing, vocational rehabilitation, crisis intervention, financial support, and advocacy. In ACT, as in the case of ICM, case managers help in discharge planning, establishing links with community programs and network to provide quality community care. ACT reduces time in the hospital and improves housing stability.

Family intervention

Call it a clan, call it a network, call it a tribe, call it a family: whatever you call it, whoever you are, you need one. Jane Howard (1935–1999)

Family involvement with the patient can have beneficial or deleterious effects on the process of recovery. Reduced rates of relapse can result from positive and effective family involvement. On the other hand, family involvement characterized by high expressed emotion (EE: hostility, criticism, overprotection) is associated with higher relapse rates. Family intervention is aimed at educational efforts and behavioral therapy focusing on preventing criticism and hostility. If EE cannot be defused, it is prudent to house the patient in an alternative setting. Furthermore, family interventions also reduce family burden and improve family well-being. Effective approaches in family intervention include empathic engagement, education, ongoing support, clinical resources during periods of crisis, social network enhancement, and problem-solving and communication skills.

Supported employment

Making a success of the job at hand is the best step toward the kind you want.
Bernard M. Baruch (1870–1965)

Most patients with schizophrenia live in the community, but frequently are socially isolated and few have jobs. Conventional approaches to vocational rehabilitation tend not to work well with patients because of the nature of the schizophrenic illness. It is more useful to identify supported worksites that are familiar with the challenges faced by patients with schizophrenia. Jobs that include flexible hours, are relatively stress-free, and offer privacy are particularly helpful. Vocational rehabilitation typically takes the approach of 'train and place' in which the training for a particular job precedes job placement. The opposite approach that uses 'place and train' has been increasingly used. It has been found that supportive employment, along with coordinated clinical care, increases the rate of competitive employment, lowers hospital admission, and improves treatment compliance. Addition of social skills training, combined with supported employment, may enhance the individual's ability to meet the interpersonal demands of the workplace.

Supported housing

The home to everyone is to him his castle and fortress, as well for his defence against injury and violence, as for his repose. Edward Coke (1553–1634)

Among the many factors that contribute to quality of life, safe and affordable housing is particularly important. The type of housing required for a patient will depend on his or her capacity to attend to housekeeping chores and general safety. Housing is an evolving 'process' in which patients initially may require a highly supervised group home setting, and over time transition to independent living. Ancillary services, such as mobile case management, crisis intervention, and continuous treatment services are often required to enable patients to be managed in the housing of their choice. Patients and clinicians often prefer this approach: quality of life is usually increased and length of hospitalizations may also be reduced.

Social skills training

Verbal and non-verbal skills that aid in communicating with others are required for socialization (the behavior patterns of the culture). These skills include the ability to hold a conversation, small talk, active listening, appropriate body language including eye contact, paying attention, and expressing interest. Social skill deficits are a hallmark of schizophrenia. Patients with schizophrenia often develop these deficits after the emergence of the illness, while some have these deficits long before the onset of psychosis. These troublesome deficits are likely due to a combination of positive and negative symptoms, and cognitive deficits, and lead to shrinking social networks and feelings of loneliness. Social skills training (SST) is a well-researched and widely used intervention. Complex social skills, such as making friends, are broken down into simpler and smaller steps and then taught using a variety of techniques, including didactic and Socratic instruction, modeling, corrective feedback, and homework exercises. SST can be conducted in individual and group sessions.

Summary

- Rehabilitation is a collection of therapeutic activities with the aim of returning the patient with schizophrenia to the highest possible level of physical, psychological, social, and environmental functioning.
- Rehabilitation is one of the three components required for recovery; pharmacological and psychosocial treatments are the other two components.
- The specific needs of a patient will determine which of the various rehabilitation methods should be employed. Typical clinical scenarios and suggested treatment approaches are listed in Table 11.1

Table 11.1 Choosing rehabilitation methods

The issue	What to do
The patient is finding it difficult to arrange a variety of appointments for follow-up, groups, pharmacy, job, etc.	Case management
The patient frequently runs out of medications and begins to worry about imminent relapse and starts calling the ambulance.	Intensive case management (ICM) or assertive community treatment (ACT)
The patient has been admitted to the inpatient service and requires housing that also supervises medication administration and follow-up with medical services for diabetes.	ACT and supported housing
The patient has been placed with his family after discharge for first episode of schizophrenia. The parents blame themselves for their son's illness. The siblings are increasingly critical because the patient does not do his 'share' of chores at home.	Family intervention and psychoeducation
The patient has been in partial remission after 1 year of treatment and now wishes to start a part-time job that primarily involves data entry. He has no means of transportation and has never worked before.	Supported employment and ICM
After 1-year duration of gradual symptom resolution the patient returns to her family, and discovers that most of her friends are no longer contacting her. She wishes to start making acquaintances, particularly males, but feels unable to do so. She has no way of getting around.	Social skills training and case management

chapter 12

Managing treatment-related complications

The worst thing about medicine is that one kind makes anther necessary.
Elbert Hubbard (1856–1915)

And it will fall out as in a complication of diseases, that by applying a remedy to one sore, you will provoke another; and that which removes the one ill symptom produces others. Sir Thomas More (1478–1535)

Complications of treatment, in the form of side effects, are so common with antipsychotic drugs (APDs) that they might as well be considered inherent to treatment. Fortunately, the majority of patients experience few and transient side effects that do not prevent continued treatment. On the other hand, there are a variety of troublesome side effects that require prompt attention in order to alleviate the discomfort. Additionally, persistent side effects are one of the commonest reasons for treatment non-adherence (see Chapter 14), which obviously increases the risk for decompensation and relapse. Therefore, one should have familiarity with expected and common side effects, as well as serious and potentially permanent complications.

General principles

The chances of a favorable outcome are improved, while also minimizing treatment-related discomfort, if the following commandments and conditions (all the Cs) are followed.

- Collaboration: establish therapeutic alliance
- Comprehensive assessment, including medication and allergy history
- Consent for treatment, following psychoeducation
- Communication: about reasons and expectations of treatment; review as often as necessary
- Communicate to the patient about the specific drug(s) to be used and expected side effects, emphasizing that most are transient
- Correct medicine for the diagnosis
- Choose the right medicine for the given set of symptoms, co-morbid conditions, and cost
- Covert concerns: inquire about side effects; sexual side effects may not be volunteered
- Convey that there are remedies for side effects and be prompt in managing them
- Contact: stay in touch with patient and family
- Complete the course of treatment (avoid switching APD prematurely)
- Compliance check
- Consultations, as needed, for second opinion or medical reasons
- Chart notes: always provide treatment rationale in progress notes
- Commiserate with patient if side effects are persistent, acknowledge the distress and frustration experienced by the patient
- Consistently, **start low, go slow** when initiating treatment.

Table 12.1 summarizes general side effects and range of severity for different body systems whereas management of common side effects is discussed in Table 12.2.

JB is a young male admitted to the hospital for severe hallucinations and aggressive behavior. He was administered 5 mg haloperidol in the Emergency Room. He presents at the nursing station in obvious distress with his tongue sticking out and eyes rolling up.

Q12.1   *What is going on?*
What remedy will you offer?

Table 12.1 APD side effects by **system**

System	Side effect	Atypical APDs	Typical APDs
Neurological	Sedation	++ – +++	High potency ±
			Low potency +++
	Acute extrapyramidal	±	High potency +++
	syndromes (EPS)		Low potency ++
	Tardive dyskinesia (TD)	± – +	+++
	Akathisia	± – +	+++
	Neuroleptic malignant	+	+
	syndrome (NMS)		
	Seizures	± – ++	High potency +
		(highest risk with clozapine)	Low potency ++
	Cognitive impairment	±	± – ++
Cardiovascular	Orthostatic hypotension	± – +++	High potency ± – +
		(highest risk with clozapine)	Low potency +++
	Electrocardiogram changes	+ – ++	+ – +++
Hematologic	Agranulocytosis	± – +++	± – ++
		(highest risk with clozapine)	
	Leukopenia and neutropenia	± – +++	High potency ±
		(highest risk with clozapine)	Low potency +++
Gastrointestinal	Nausea	± – ++	± – ++
	Constipation	± – +++	High potency ±
		(highest risk with clozapine)	Low potency +++
	Hepatotoxicity	++	++
Neuroendocrine	Hyperprolactinemia	± – ++	+++
	Sexual dysfunction	± – ++	± – ++
	Weight gain	± – +++	± – ++
		(highest risk with olanzapine and clozapine)	
	Dyslipidemias	± – +++	± – +
		(highest risk with olanzapine and clozapine)	
	Diabetes mellitus	± – +++	± – +
		(highest risk with olanzapine and clozapine)	
Genitourinary	Urinary incontinence	± – +++	± – ++
		(highest risk with clozapine)	
Dermatologic	Photosensitivity	±	High potency ±
			Low potency +++

± = none to minimal; + = mild; ++ = moderate; +++ = marked

Table 12.2 Management of side effects arranged in alphabetical order

Treatment-related problem	*What to do*
Agranulocytosis Granulocyte count falls below 500/mm³ leading to heightened risk of fatal infections	While most commonly associated with clozapine, it can occur with any APD. It is a life-threatening side effect. Agranulocytosis is a medical emergency that requires hospitalization, isolation, prophylactic antibiotics, granulocyte colony-stimulating factor and granulocyte-macrophage colony stimulating factor
Akathisia Subjective feeling of motor restlessness (jitteriness) felt mostly in the legs, and discomfort. Usually seen early in treatment	Lower the dose of APD. Akathisia is not responsive to anticholinergic drugs; beta-blockers like propranolol are more effective. Benzodiazepines can also be helpful. Since akathisia is most commonly observed with typical APDs, switching to atypical APDs, other than high doses of risperidone, may offer the best solution
Anorgasmia Inability to achieve orgasm. It is more prevalent in women	This is not reported frequently in spite of being relatively common. Therefore, it is important to ask specifically about sexual side effects. Lowering the dose or changing the APD can be helpful. Sildenafil has been used successfully in antidepressant-induced anorgasmia
Blurred vision	The most common reason for blurred vision is anticholinergic effect of some APDs. If these APDs cannot be avoided, then pilocarpine or bethanecol may be used
Constipation	A common problem due to anticholinergic effects, low fiber intake and immobility. It can be treated with increased fiber intake (bran, vegetables and fruits, psyllium), prunes, increased non-calorie fluid intake, stool softeners (docusate) and exercise. Laxatives should be used sparingly
Dry mouth (xerostomia; *xero*, **dry)**	It is due to anticholinergic effects of APDs. Switch to an alternative APD if possible. Otherwise, advise chewing sugar-free gum, sips of cold calorie-free fluids or ice chips. Pilocarpine rinse may be helpful

Dysphoria
A feeling of unpleasantness, unease, emotional discomfort

Dysphoria can be a consequence of treatment, though patients find it difficult to describe, and clinicians frequently ignore it or attribute it to the illness. Changes in treatment on the basis of this complaint should be made cautiously because dysphoria can be part of the illness. However, trial lowering of the dose is worthwhile, or switching the APD

Dystonia
Acute painful contraction of muscles, usually affecting the tongue, neck, eyes and trunk leading to protruding tongue, abnormal head position, grimacing, eyes rolling up and neck spasm

Initially treat with intramuscular or intravenous benztropine 2 mg or diphenhydramine 50 mg; repeat after 15 minutes if no response. Usually there is prompt and dramatic relief. Thereafter, continue oral anticholinergic treatment. Dystonia frequency has been reduced by increasing use of atypical APDs

Ejaculatory dysfunction
Delayed or inability to ejaculate, or retrograde ejaculation

Reduced dose of APD can be effective. Alternatively, switch to atypical APD

Erectile dysfunction
inability to achieve and maintain a penile erection

Lowering the dose or changing the APD can be helpful. Sildenafil and analogs have been used successfully in antidepressant-induced erectile dysfunction

Glucose metabolism abnormality
Abnormal glucose tolerance test result, increased fasting glucose levels or frank diabetes mellitus

Impaired glucose tolerance, hyperglycemia and diabetes mellitus are observed primarily with atypical APDs, particularly clozapine and olanzapine. Management includes switching APD, monitoring glucose levels, weight loss if indicated, and hypoglycemic agents if diabetes mellitus develops

Hyperprolactinemia
Elevation of prolactin above 20 µg/l, caused by dopamine blockade. Chronic prolactin elevation can cause amenorrhea, galactorrhea, gynecomastia, and possible loss of bone density

With the availability of atypical APDs with low propensity to induce hyperprolactinemia, it is wiser to switch APDs rather than attempting treatment with dopamine agonists such as cyproheptadine

Hyperthermia

Mild elevation of body temperature which is common during initial treatment, particularly with clozapine, can be treated with antipyretics. Persistent hyperthermia

Table 12.2 continued

Treatment-related problem	What to do
	or higher temperatures can be indicative of serious conditions and should be promptly investigated
Leukopenia Decrease in white blood cells, generally ≤4000 to 5000 cells/mm³	It is usually transient but requires careful watching with repeated white blood counts because it may be a harbinger of agranulocytosis
Libido decrease	Decreased libido can occur in 25–50% of patients. Switching APDs can reverse such libido reduction
Lipid abnormalities Desirable cholesterol level <200 mg/dl Triglyceride level <150 mg/dl	Elevations in triglyceride and cholesterol levels occur with atypical APDs, particularly clozapine and olanzapine. The degree of elevations is not well correlated with weight gain. If switching to another APD is not feasible, conservative measures (weight loss, exercise, dietary changes) and lipid-lowering agents should be used
Liver enzyme elevation Alanine transaminase range 15–45 U/l	Increases in liver enzymes, particularly transaminases, are common and transient. In the event of persistent elevations or clinical hepatotoxicity, prompt referral to gastroenterologist is required
Neutropenia Decrease in neutrophils, <2000 cells/mm³	It occurs in about 20% of patients treated with clozapine, and is usually transient
Neuroleptic malignant syndrome NMS, is sudden onset of muscle rigidity and hyperthermia, along with altered consciousness, autonomic instability, and elevations in white blood cells and creatine phosphokinase (CPK)	NMS is potentially fatal and can occur with practically all APDs. If NMS is suspected, assess promptly. If confirmed, immediately stop the APD, and start supportive treatment (hydration, lower body temperature, correct electrolyte imbalance). Dopamine *agonists* (e.g. bromocriptine) or dantrolene may be used. After recovery, a different APD should be introduced cautiously

Orthostatic hypotension
Fall in blood pressure occurring while arising from a seated or lying position accompanied by faintness and light-headedness

Generally transient, rarely lasting longer than 4–6 weeks. Commonsense measures include advice about standing up slowly, getting out of bed slowly, elevating the headrest, increase fluids and salt intake. If conservative measures fail, fludrocortisone may be tried. *Epinephrine* is contraindicated

Parkinsonism
Tremor, rigidity, bradykinesia (slow movements) and shuffling gait

Most commonly seen with typical APDs. Dose reduction along with anticholinergic agents (e.g. benztropine) is generally quite effective. Alternatively, switch to atypical APD

Q–Tc prolongation
The QT interval, the duration of ventricular depolarization and repolarization, is normally 380–420 ms. QT prolongation >500 ms is associated with the development of cardiac dysrhythmias, particularly *torsades de pointes* that can lead to sudden death

Clearly, careful cardiac monitoring should be instituted with increased Q–Tc interval, particularly in those individuals with a medical history that is suggestive of heart disease. It is best to switch APDs to those less likely to induce Q–Tc prolongation

Rabbit syndrome
Involuntary perioral tremor that mimics a rabbit chewing, arises late in treatment

Unlike other late onset (tardive) motor disorders associated with APDs that don't respond to anticholinergic treatment, the rabbit syndrome responds well to benztropine or other anticholinergic agents

Sedation

In most instances sedation is transient and lasts about 2 weeks. When it interferes with functioning, change the dosing to all at bedtime, reduce daytime dosing and, if unsuccessful, switch to a less sedating APD

Seizures

Usually occur with rapid escalation of APD dose, and in a dose-dependent manner with clozapine. In the case of clozapine divided dosing may decrease the risk. Anticonvulsants may need to be used

Sialorrhea
Drooling or excessive salivation is the pooling of saliva beyond the margin of the lip. Common with clozapine and it is not transient

Patients find sialorrhea quite bothersome. It tends to worsen during sleep. A towel over the pillow can help with the physical discomfort. Anticholinergic agents have been used with success

Table 12.2 continued

Treatment-related problem	What to do
Tachycardia Rapid heartbeat >100 beats/min	It tends to be a transient side effect, seen with APDs with higher anticholinergicity or due to orthostatic hypotension. If persistent, atenolol may be used
Tardive dyskinesia (TD) Non-rhythmic choreiform (jerky) or athetoid (slow writhing) movements typically affecting the tongue, lips, jaw, fingers, toes, and trunk. TD can be transient or permanent	There is no definitive treatment for TD. Stopping the APD, and switching to an atypical APD is likely to provide significant relief over the course of several months or longer. Transient worsening of TD can occur when the APD dose is reduced. Clozapine is effective in some cases of severe and persistent TD. The role of vitamin E in treating and preventing TD has not been resolved
Weight gain Body mass index (BMI) is weight in kilograms ÷ height in m² Normal BMI: 18.5–24.9 Overweight: 25–29.9 Obese: >30	APDs vary significantly in their effect on weight. Because atypical APDs are increasingly used as first-line treatment, weight gain with these drugs has garnered most attention. Clozapine and olanzapine have the highest weight gain potential, while ziprasidone has the least. It is prudent to initiate weight management principles concurrently with treatment, which include education, nutritional counseling, exercise, lifestyle alterations. If these measures fail, then switch APD if clinically feasible. Controlling weight gain during treatment is a significant challenge because it occurs within the context of a larger societal problem of increasing obesity

Metabolic syndrome

Metabolic syndrome, also called syndrome X or insulin resistance syndrome, deserves special mention because patients with schizophrenia appear to be at increased risk for developing it, and the risk is significantly heightened with the use of APDs, particularly clozapine and olanzapine. The metabolic syndrome is associated with increased risk of type 2 diabetes mellitus (DM) and coronary heart disease, stroke, and peripheral vascular disease.

Metabolic syndrome is the clustering of specific risk factors for cardiovascular disease and type 2 DM that occur together in the same individual. The definition of the metabolic syndrome varies somewhat, but the most widely accepted is the Adult Treatment Panel III criteria (from the third report of the US National Cholesterol Education Program expert panel on Detection, Evaluation, and Treatment of High Blood Cholesterol in Adults). Specifically, the presence of **three or more** of the following components defines the metabolic syndrome:

Central obesity (fat tissue in and around the abdomen) as measured by waist circumference (men > 40 inches (100 cm); women > 35 inches (87 cm))

Fasting blood triglycerides ≥ 150 mg/dl

Blood HDL ('good') cholesterol (men < 40 mg/dl; women < 50 mg/dl)

Blood pressure ≥ 130/85 mmHg

Fasting glucose ≥ 110 mg/dl

The causes of this syndrome are genetic factors, overweight/obesity and physical inactivity, probably mediated through the effects of insulin resistance (when the body can't properly use insulin to move glucose into cells).

Since metabolic syndrome comprises multiple risk factors, treatment **WILL** have to be multi-pronged and progress assessed frequently.

Weight loss

Increase physical activity

Lower blood pressure

Lower glucose and lipid levels

Diabetes

One of the consequences of metabolic syndrome is DM. The relationship between diabetes and schizophrenia is an interesting one. An association between diabetes and psychosis was noted as early as the 1890s, and patients with schizophrenia have twice the prevalence rates of DM than the general population. The concern about DM has risen with the introduction of APDs, and most recently because of the increasing use of atypical APDs that are associated with substantial weight gain, such as olanzapine and clozapine. Once DM is diagnosed or pre-existing DM worsens, the standard treatment for DM should be instituted, along with switching to a less diabetogenic APD.

ANSWERS

Q12.1 JB is presenting with classic acute dystonia, with protruding tongue and oculogyric crisis (eyes locked upwards). Other presentations include spasms of the neck and trunk. Even laryngospasm can occur with breathing difficulties. Prompt treatment with intramuscular or intravenous benztropine 2 mg or diphenhydramine 50 mg; repeat after 10–15 minutes if no response. Usually there is prompt and dramatic relief. In those individuals at risk (young, male, high dose of typical APD) oral anticholinergic may be used prophylactically. Atypical APDs are a better choice in high-risk individuals.

chapter 13

Suboptimal treatment response

In a certain sense every drug a doctor administers and every operation a surgeon performs is experimental in that the result can never be mathematically calculated, the doctor's judgment and the patient's response being variables indeterminable by any law of averages.

Harvey Cushing (1869–1939)

A 46-year-old woman has been treated with 40 mg olanzapine daily for 2 months, after the failure of 8 mg of risperidone for 3 months to reduce the severity of hallucinations. The patient is demoralized at the lack of response to the current regimen and wants to alter treatment.

What are the next steps in managing the illness?

Q13.1   Order the sequence of steps:
1. Increase dose of olanzapine
2. Add a typical antipsychotic
3. Start clozapine
4. Assess treatment compliance
5. Check for substance abuse
6. Reassess diagnosis
7. Inquire about stressors

What is suboptimal treatment response?

When treatment fails to provide satisfactory resolution of the symptoms of schizophrenia, it is important to first ask whether *optimal* treatment is being provided.

Optimal pharmacotherapy can be thought of as the appropriate drug at an adequate dose for an adequate length of time with the least burden of side effects and treatment complexity.

One-third of patients with schizophrenia, unfortunately, do not respond satisfactorily to optimal treatment. It is important to note that satisfactory response does not mean the absence of *all* signs and symptoms of schizophrenia. In fact, treatment that achieves symptom resolution to meet criteria for the residual subtype (page 47, Tables 5.4) would be considered an excellent therapeutic response.

Researchers utilize a variety of criteria of treatment response, focused usually on the reduction of positive symptoms (hallucinations, delusions and thought disorder) as assessed by rating scales, such as the commonly used Brief Psychiatric Rating Scale (BPRS). For example, a common criterion of treatment response in research studies is 50% reduction of positive symptoms, as rated on the BPRS, by the end of the study. This does represent a substantial reduction in symptom severity from baseline, but is not informative about the adequacy of treatment response for a particular patient. Fifty per cent reduction in positive symptoms can still leave a patient with many troublesome symptoms.

At a practical level the estimation of therapeutic response in an individual patient is dependent on a combination of factors, such as reduction of most symptoms, acceptance of some residual symptoms, and the tolerability of treatment.

BR is 38 years old and married, with long-standing schizophrenia. He is being treated with 20 mg of olanzapine. He has put on 15 kg (30 lb) in weight. The auditory hallucinations are infrequent. He remains uncomfortable in crowds, but is able to commute to the job center where he does simple tasks for a stipend.

Would you change his treatment – yes or no?

Q13.2   If yes, why would you change it?
1. He still has auditory hallucinations
2. He has had weight gain
3. He is uncomfortable in crowds
4. He can only do simple tasks
5. The dose of olanzapine is too high

Response to treatment occurs along a continuum, ranging from no response at all to a rapid, complete and sustained resolution of symptoms. Most patients have a treatment response that falls somewhere between the two extremes (Figure 13.1).

No response	Treatment refractory	Treatment resistance*	Partial response	Response	Complete recovery
No change in any aspect of illness with optimal treatment	Persistence of positive symptoms in spite of two or more adequate trials with antipsychotic drugs	Persistence of positive symptoms with optimal treatment	Reduction of symptoms, but persistence of some positive symptoms	Significant reduction of symptoms with improved functional capacity	Absence of all symptoms and return to baseline level of functioning

*An unfortunate term suggesting that it is the patient who is resisting treatment, which may not be the case.

Figure 13.1 The treatment response continuum.

Causes for inadequate treatment response

CY is 33 years old, with recent-onset olfactory hallucinations, periods of fear and religious preoccupation. He has been treated with 4 mg of risperidone for 2 months. Although he has been compliant with treatment, there has been no significant improvement in symptom severity.

What are your next steps?

Q13.3   What would you do?

1. Increase the dose of risperidone
2. Change the antipsychotic
3. Review the diagnosis
4. Refer to a neurologist
5. Stay the course for another month

Right diagnosis? Right medication?   In order for treatment to work, the prescribed medication needs to be appropriate for the condition in question. In other words, the treatment has to be appropriate for the patient's diagnosis. One caveat, however, has to be borne in mind. Many medications, especially the atypical antipsychotic drugs, have beneficial effects across a variety of diagnostic categories; for example, all the atypical antipsychotic drugs have been shown to have therapeutic effects in the mood spectrum disorders as well. However, these medications are also widely prescribed in practice for conditions for which there is no evidence of antipsychotic efficacy such as autism spectrum disorders, anxiety, post-traumatic stress disorders, and so forth. The clinician therefore has to first ask the question whether the diagnosis is right, while considering reasons for treatment resistance.

CR is a 26-year-old single mother with 3 young children who has been prescribed Geodon 40 mg BID, clozapine 50 mg BID, depakote 500 mg q AM and 250 mg at noon, 500 mg q HS and benztropine 1 mg BID. The severity of delusions of reference remains unchanged.

Q13.4 What would you do?
1. Increase the dose of clozapine
2. Check the depakote levels
3. Inquire about compliance
4. Inquire about the children's health
5. Offer hospitalization

Was the medication taken by the patient?   Even if the diagnosis and the prescribed treatment are correct, the patient may not be taking the medication as prescribed. The most common reason for this is treatment non-adherence. The factors that lead to non-adherence and approaches to address them are detailed in Chapter 14.

CR, the patient described above, has had her treatment regimen simplified. She is now taking clozapine 200 mg BID and depakote 500 mg BID. The delusions of reference are less bothersome, but she complains of not getting enough sleep and is losing weight.

Q13.5 What would you do?
1. Increase the dose of clozapine
2. Check the depakote levels
3. Inquire about compliance
4. Inquire about the children's health
5. Inquire about her support system

Are psychosocial stressors compromising treatment response?   In spite of seemingly optimal treatment there can be suboptimal response. After re-assessing diagnosis and compliance, it is prudent to ask about stressors in a patient's life. It is well known that stress can increase the risk for decompensation and relapse. Likewise, stress can compromise ongoing treatment. It is important not to assume that situations not ordinarily stressful to you or I would not be stressful to a patient. Addressing specific psychosocial stressors (stress reduction) can be very helpful for the overall outcome as well as improving specific treatment response.

Does the drug have optimum concentration in the body? Even when the medication prescribed is taken with good compliance there are other reasons why adequate concentrations may not have been reached. Plasma concentrations depend on both the rate of dosing of a medication as well as its clearance by the body, generally by liver enzymes – cytochrome oxidases. The metabolic rate of a given drug may vary from person to person; some individuals metabolize at a faster rate (rapid metabolizers), others at a slower rate (slow metabolizers). At a given dose, rapid metabolizers will have lower plasma levels than slow metabolizers. Genetic factors, as well as physiological parameters (age, co-morbid illness, concurrent medications, diet and pregnancy), can affect the pharmacokinetics of medications, leading to alterations in plasma concentrations, even when the dose is constant.

Examining plasma levels of drugs has been utilized to aid proper dosing. This practice was much more common during the era of typical antipsychotic drugs (such as haloperidol). Today, the estimation of plasma levels of clozapine is most common (levels above 350 ng/ml are associated with therapeutic response). In routine practice, however, monitoring of antipsychotic drug plasma levels is not very useful.

Did the drug have the desired effect? Another factor in determining therapeutic response is that the desired effect of the drug at specific receptors in the brain is not occurring in spite of adequate plasma concentrations. There are multiple reasons for lack of effect. Individual genetic differences in receptor affinities may exist, similar to genetic differences in drug metabolism. It turns out that many of the same factors that affect pharmacokinetics noted above can affect receptor responsivity to the drug. There is much ongoing research aimed at identifying these genetic variations in order to tailor treatments to the individual patient.

Approaches to suboptimal treatment response

'*What do we do when nothing works?*' is a common lament that all practicing clinicians will have to contend with when treating patients with schizophrenia.

Because the causes of suboptimal treatment response are not always apparent, or even discoverable, the practical approach to managing this is one of empiricism (Greek *empeiria*, meaning experience). Clinical experience and observation, supported by available research evidence (evidence-based practice), should guide the treatment.

> Before embarking on empirical modification of treatment, review once again for the presence of factors associated with suboptimal treatment response (diagnosis, substance abuse, co-morbid disorders, and psychosocial stressors).

Raise the dose. This was common practice in the 1970s and 1980s, the so-called high dose and rapid neuroleptization strategies which led to serious extrapyramidal complications while using typical antipsychotic drugs. The general thinking used to be that if you double the dose you would have double the effect. However, keep in mind that if a medication is ineffective for other reasons, raising the dose is unlikely to help, and will only increase the risk of side effects. With that in mind, however, recent studies of antipsychotic drugs have suggested that previous estimates of the optimum doses are being revised. For example, the initial recommended dose for quetiapine was an underestimate and studies indicate better efficacy with higher doses. This is true of olanzapine as well. On the other hand, the initial recommended dose for risperidone was too high and had to be revised downward. The key concept to consider is achieving a minimum effective dose, that is, a dose that is effective but not high enough to cause side effects.

Lower the dose or try without it. Higher doses than recommended may diminish efficacy, because of side effects, and the wiser step may be to reduce the dose. For example, treating akathisia by lowering the antipsychotic dose can have salutary effects on psychosis severity. When there is lack of clarity it may be worth considering a brief period off medication. Such medication-free trials carry significant risk of further worsening of the patient's condition and need to be conducted in carefully controlled settings, such as the inpatient service.

Add another medication. It is a common practice to add either another antipsychotic or mood stabilizer to an existing antipsychotic medication. While polypharmacy is generally not recommended, it may be useful to consider medication combinations, especially if the benefits are complementary and there are no additive side effects. For example, it is unwise to combine two medications both of which have similar side effects such as weight gain, for example olanzapine and quetiapine; on the other hand combining a highly sedative antipsychotic such as clozapine with an activating antipsychotic such as aripiprazole may be worth considering in specific situations.

Switch to a new medication. If the current antipsychotic medication is convincingly ineffective this is an appropriate approach. By and large it is better to consider interclass as opposed to intraclass switching of the medications. For example, it would make little sense to switch from trifluoperazine to perphenazine, both of which are phenothiazines. On the other hand it may be worth considering to switch from a typical to an atypical antipsychotic drug. If two or more antipsychotic medications have been found ineffective, the appropriate next step is to consider clozapine if there are no contraindications. Clozapine is not a benign drug, however, and has serious side effects that would require monitoring for hematological complications.

Summary

- **Suboptimal treatment response** is when treatment fails to provide satisfactory resolution of the symptoms. One-third of patients with schizophrenia do not respond satisfactorily to optimal treatment.
- The assessment of therapeutic response in an individual patient is dependent on a combination of factors such as reduction of the most symptoms, acceptance of some residual symptoms, and the tolerability of treatment.
- Response to treatment occurs along a continuum, ranging from no response at all to a rapid, complete and sustained resolution of symptoms.
- Questions to ask in the case of suboptimal treatment response are:
  - Right diagnosis? Right medication?
  - Was the medication taken by the patient?
  - Are psychosocial stressors compromising treatment response?
  - Does the drug have optimum concentration in the body?
  - Did the drug have the desired effect?
- **Causes of suboptimal treatment response** are not always apparent, or even discoverable. Therefore, an empirical approach is required, informed by research evidence (summarized in Figure 13.1).

- Raise the dose
- Lower the dose or try without it
- Add another medication
- Switch to a new medication

ANSWERS

Q13.1 Our recommendation would be the following sequence of steps:
1. Reassess diagnosis
2. Assess treatment compliance
3. Check for substance abuse
4. Inquire about stressors
5. Start clozapine
6. Add a typical antipsychotic

We would not recommend increasing the dose of olanzapine.

Q13.2 It is unlikely we would change BR's treatment at this time because he appears to be doing fairly well. However, we would consider changing treatment if the patient expresses concern about the weight gain, discomfort with crowds, or cognitive deficits that prevent advancement in his job. If the concern is limited to the infrequent auditory hallucinations, we would carefully review the

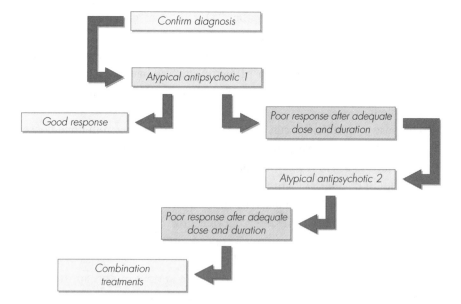

Figure 13.1 A typical treatment algorithm.

advantages of tolerating residual symptoms and the disadvantages of altering a fairly effective treatment regimen, urging that treatment not be changed at this time.

Q13.3 In addition to reviewing the history of the illness, we would refer CY to a neurologist in order to assess for a seizure disorder. The recent-onset olfactory hallucinations, periods of fear and religious preoccupation are consistent with temporal lobe epilepsy, the treatment of which requires antiepileptic agents. Risperidone may need to be continued to treat any residual psychosis. Antipsychotic drugs that lower the seizure threshold, such as clozapine, should be avoided.

Q13.4 CR has been prescribed a complicated regimen. The persistence of symptoms may indicate non-adherence with treatment. Missing or forgetting medications is an extremely common occurrence. The more complicated the medication regimen, the greater likelihood of missing a dose. The first task would be to simplify CR's medication regimen by following the **KISS** principle of pharmacotherapy (Keep it **S**afe & **S**imple).

Q13.5 CR appears to be responding to treatment, following the simplification of the treatment regimen and improved compliance. The inadequate sleep and weight loss may be new concerns or old concerns coming to light with the reduction in psychosis. Before considering any change in treatment, it is important to determine whether she's experiencing stress, a well-known cause of sleep and appetite disturbance. CR is a single mother with three young children. The absence of social supports or ill health in children can easily lead to increased stress, which can increase the risk of psychotic relapse.

chapter 14

Treatment non-adherence

How can we assure ourselves of his convalescence, and prevent relapses, if the patient is not submitted during a period, more or less protracted, to a mode of life appropriate to his constitution, and to the causes and character of the malady from which he has just been restoreds ... if he is not watchful against errors of regimen, excess of study, and transports of passion?

Jean-Etienne Dominique Esquirol (1772–1840)

Arguably one of the greatest challenges that a clinician will face in caring for the patient with schizophrenia is non-adherence to treatment. There are a multitude of reasons why patients don't comply with treatment. Regardless of the reason, the result of non-adherence can be devastating to patients and their families.

Most clinicians underestimate treatment non-adherence

(Nearly three-quarters of patients become non-adherent within 2 years following discharge.)

It is paramount that the possibility of non-adherence be taken into account from initial treatment contact. Non-compliance is more common early in the course of schizophrenia. Denial of the illness is the most common cause.

General principles

What is adherence?

Simply, treatment adherence or compliance is taking medicine as prescribed by the physician, including the dose, timing, frequency, and duration specified. Treatment adherence also includes prescribed prohibitions, such as avoiding alcohol and illicit drugs, driving or operating machinery, and avoiding specified foods or other substances. Any deviation from the prescribed regimen constitutes non-adherence.

How common is non-adherence?

Given the above definition, you would correctly surmise that treatment non-adherence is relatively common across all medical specialties (Figure 14.1), but more so in persons with schizophrenia.

Why does non-adherence matter?

The consequences of non-adherence depend on its nature. Partial non-adherence can result in incomplete treatment response, increase the risk of chronicity as well as relapse. With total non-adherence, relapse is virtually certain.

How do we assess non-adherence?

Since both clinicians and patients underestimate non-adherence, it is useful practice, particularly early in treatment, to rely on objective and practical methods to estimate treatment adherence, such as pill count. We recommend asking patients

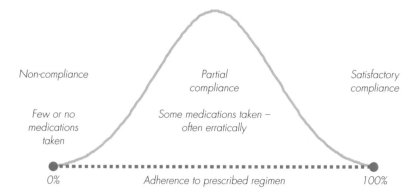

Non-compliance

Few or no medications taken

Partial compliance

Some medications taken – often erratically

Satisfactory compliance

0%   *Adherence to prescribed regimen*   *100%*

Figure 14.1 Degree of non-adherence.

to bring their pill bottles with them during outpatient visits. It is also very useful to inquire about adherence from family members or support staff.

Suspect non-adherence when you note:

- unexplained change in behavior
- missed appointments
- evidence of substance abuse (smell of alcohol on breath, pupils that are dilated or pinpoint)
- the patient is beginning a new relationship – inquire especially about sexual side effects and the partner's views about medications and mental illness.

What causes non-adherence?

There are many reasons why patients choose not to comply with treatment as prescribed. Early in the course of illness, denial of illness is one of the commonest reasons. Medication side effects are another very common reason. Figure 14.2 provides a dimensional view of the causes of treatment non-adherence.

> *When faced with treatment non-adherence, each of the above factors must be taken into account. In fact, astute clinicians always keep these factors in mind when interacting with patients.*

How do we manage non-adherence?

Management of treatment non-adherence depends on the factors that are operative in specific clinical situations, some of which are illustrated below. Strategies to address non-adherence can be *proactive* or *reactive* or both.

Proactive approaches are based on the fact that non-adherence occurs at very high rates, and that it is generally underestimated by both clinicians and patients. However, being proactive should not interfere with establishing therapeutic alliance – it should not be viewed as mistrust of the patient's intentions. **Reactive** approaches are instituted in the face of clear evidence of non-adherence.

An overarching set of principles in approaching treatment non-adherence has been articulated by Dr Xavier Amador (*I Am Not Sick: I Don't Need Help*, Vida Press, 2000). He calls it **LEAP** (Listen, Empathize, Agree, and Partner).

Additionally, common approaches to managing non-adherence include:

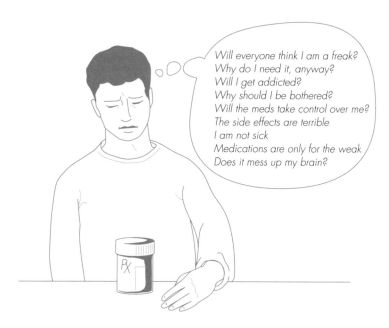

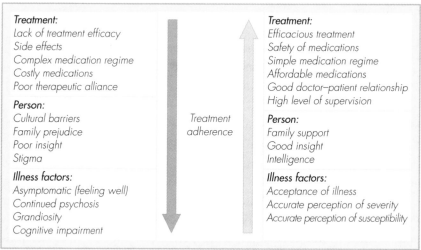

Figure 14.2 The Health Belief Model (modified from Perkins, 1999).

- *Lack of insight* is a prelude to non-adherence and withdrawal from treatment – assess insight early and proactively institute plans to engage patient in treatment; invite assistance from family and friends.
- *Improved treatment outcome.* Suboptimal therapeutic response is associated with high degrees of non-adherence. Patients can be unrealistic about

rapidity of response or presence of residual symptoms. Realign their expectations so as to be consistent with general clinical experience.

- *Side effects.* Proactively ask about side effects at each visit. Pay particular attention to sexual and cognitive side effects, and treatment-related dysphoria.
- *Simplify the treatment regimen.* Whenever possible, utilize bedtime or morning dosing, and preferably once daily. Ask patients about their preference.
- *Reduce cost of medications*, if this is an issue.
- *Inquire about cultural, religious, or social barriers* to treatment adherence.
- *Inquire about family attitudes towards psychiatric medications.* Not infrequently, families discourage any association with psychiatry, leading to non-adherence by the patient.
- *Feeling well.* Not surprisingly, patients who are recovered feel they no longer need treatment. This is the time to be vigilant: education regarding the risk of relapse without treatment must be reinforced.
- *Grandiosity or florid psychosis.* When allying with the patient's delusions to engage in treatment fails, then coercive treatments may be required if dangerousness to the patient or others is unequivocally present.

Common clinical scenarios

AC is a 31-year-old engineer who presents at the ER with a recent worsening of paranoia. He is prescribed 2 mg risperidone and discharged. He is not seen again at the outpatient clinic, but presents at the emergency room the following day believing he has 'meningitis.'

Q14.1 Why is the patient complaining about 'meningitis'? What management would you suggest?

MK is a 28-year-old man discharged from the inpatient unit on Friday. On Monday, nurses noted that he forgot to take his follow-up instructions. He missed his appointment on Wednesday, but showed up a year later with a severe psychotic decompensation.

Q14.2 Why did he miss his appointment?
If you could go back in time, what would you do?

BA is a 26-year-old woman with three young children who has been prescribed ziprasidone 40 mg BID, clozapine 50 mg BID, depakote 500 mg q AM and 750 mg q HS and benztropine 1 mg BID. One day, the police are called mid-day since she does not answer her door and the children are crying inside.

Q14.3 What do you think happened?
How would you manage this medication regimen?

JL, a 21-year-old college freshman, is admitted for 'odd' behavior after trying to climb the science building, and patrolling the neighborhood at night so that he can save lives. He does not believe he is ill, and refuses all medications.

Q14.4 Why do you think JL is refusing medications?
How would you get him to take medicines?

STRONG FEELINGS! Patients who refuse medications often generate strong feelings in treating staff. This stems from a sense of helplessness at not being able to bear upon a 'helpless' patient to comply with treatment, as well as feelings of anger at the patient for not 'cooperating'. While these feelings may appear understandable, they have the power to unconsciously distort relations with the patient in unhelpful ways. It is imperative that clinicians remind themselves that a patient who refuses treatment has an illness that underlies the behavior. This reframe on a patient's 'obstinate' behavior allows proactive and empathetic actions for and on his or her behalf.

KC is a 34-year-old unemployed lawyer treated with olanzapine 40 mg daily for intractable beliefs that his family has been replaced by 'replicas'. The clinician during re-evaluation is puzzled that he has not put on any weight.

Q14.5 What are the key points to consider here?
How would you facilitate treatment adherence?

Long-acting depot antipsychotic agents

All currently available long-acting depot antipsychotics are administered intramuscularly. Therein lies the trouble that patients and clinicians have with regard to using them.

Patients often view the suggestion for using depot antipsychotics quite negatively because it may indicate to them that:

- they are not to be trusted in complying with oral medications
- the patient is a 'tough' case and requires more 'serious' treatment
- the doctor (and often society, by extension) is taking away his or her liberty to refuse treatment or choose the kind of treatment
- the doctor wants to punish the patient.

These concerns of patients have to be taken seriously. Remember that depot antipsychotics are no panacea either. After all, a patient may submit to one injection of the depot, but later refuse to return to the clinic altogether! However, depot antipsychotics do offer a variety of advantages:

- patients receive prescribed doses
- predictable and stable plasma concentrations
- efficacy with lower doses
- no risk of abrupt discontinuation
- rapid identification of non-adherence.

Summary

Table 14.1 Strategies for managing treatment non-adherence

The problem	What to do
Patient refuses medications	Improve therapeutic alliance; rapid acting medications; involuntary medications as last resort
Patient is non-adherent because medications are not working	Dosage adjustment; consider medication switch, clozapine
Patient is non-adherent because of side effects	Dosage adjustment; consider medication switch; monitor & educate regarding side effects
Patient does not show up for first appointment	Improve hospital-to-clinic continuity; make care more accessible and patient-friendly
Patient who frequently misses/ forgets medications or appointments	Cues to remember; memory aids such as pillboxes and alarm watches; phone call reminders; depot medication
Patient believes he/she does not need medications	Compliance therapy; continuing psychoeducation; cognitive remediation

ANSWERS

Q14.1 AC was experiencing motor side effects (extrapyramidal side effects, particularly neck rigidity). Management includes lowering antipsychotic drug dose, treating the side effects with anticholinergic agents, and switching antipsychotic, if possible, to one that has a lower propensity for motor side effects.

Side effects are a very common reason for non-adherence. The clinician should be familiar with the usual side effects of medications they prescribe, and communicate these to the patient with sensitivity and reassurance. Family members should also be informed of side effects so that they can help monitor the patient, particularly during the early days of treatment.

Q14.2 MK did not show up for his appointment likely because no therapeutic alliance was established prior to discharge and aggressive follow-up care was not instituted. To facilitate aftercare, therapeutic continuity should be enhanced, barriers to treatment should be assessed, and letters should be written if phone contact is unsuccessful.

Patients miss appointments for many reasons, but a common one is lack of alliance with the clinician. It is vital that the patient be a partner in his or her care. This minimizes the possibility of non-adherence. Patients who appear not to care about their treatment should be closely monitored. While there are 'passive' patients who go along with treatment, they can just as easily slip out of treatment.

Q14.3 BA either was not taking medication as prescribed and decompensated or accidentally overdosed. What BA needs is a simpler medication regimen (KISS – *Keep it Safe and Simple*). Any barriers to taking medications should be identified and cues developed for taking medication. Tracking compliance, for example by checking refill dates or pill counting, can help the clinician intervene early.

Missing or forgetting medications is an extremely common occurrence in all of medicine, but particularly so in psychiatry. The more complicated the medication regimen, the greater the likelihood of missing a dose. Just as concerning with a complicated medication regimen is the risk of overdosing. Imagine a scenario in which an otherwise diligent patient has to contend with three different medications over four different time points daily. Simplify, simplify and simplify!

Q14.4 JL has no insight into the nature of his behavior or its consequences. First, actively listen to JL's concerns. This may help him feel understood and possibly improve the chances of JL listening to you in return! Elicit support from family and friends who may be able to influence his decisions. Obtain a second opinion if necessary. As a last resort, initiate the process for compulsory medication only if JL is a danger to himself or others

Patients who refuse medications because they lack insight into the nature or severity of their illness are especially challenging to persuade to partner in their care. Every effort should be made to get them to initiate treatment. Sometimes short-acting antianxiety agents can reduce the severity of the illness to permit negotiation regarding antipsychotic medications. Although there is a continuum of opinions regarding forced treatment, always bear in mind that any intervention must be in the patient's best interest.

Q14.5 It appears that the treatment offered has not been effective. Since olanzapine is associated with some weight gain, its absence raises the possibility of non-adherence. Thus, assess compliance: if KC has been compliant with treatment, then titrate the olanzapine dose and ensure an adequate duration of treatment; if still no response, attempt augmentation strategies or change the antipsychotic prescribed.

Epilog

Patients are sometimes non-adherent because treatment is not effective. The presence of unacceptable side effects can increase the likelihood of non-adherence in the face of poor treatment response. Partial or non-response is a clinical reality. The trick is to maintain the patient's (and your) hopes that a better response will be forthcoming with better dosing or alternative treatments. The key, we believe, is in positive engagement with the patient and active listening to his or her concerns.

chapter 15

Managing decompensation and relapse

When life kicks you, let it kick you forward. Eli Stanley Jones (1884–1972)

Schizophrenia has to be treated lifelong. This does *not* mean that individuals with schizophrenia cannot have good recovery with a high quality of life. However, for many patients the course of illness is beset with episodes of decompensation and relapse. The challenge for the patient and clinician is to minimize the frequency and severity of relapse. It is well known that each episode of relapse becomes harder to treat than the previous one.

Decompensation We define decompensation as clinical worsening from current level of stability that does not meet criteria for relapse; it is transitory and fluid. The clinical worsening can spontaneously return to previous level of stability without active intervention or progress to a relapsed state. We find it useful to distinguish decompensation from relapse; it allows us to track clinical changes that merit careful monitoring.

Relapse While there are a variety of research criteria for relapse (e.g. 25% worsening from baseline), in general it is understood as clinical worsening that requires active intervention, ranging from adjustment of antipsychotic drug (APD) dose to hospitalization.

Prediction of relapse

Early in the course of illness it can be difficult to predict the likelihood of relapse. The clinician is likely to be on firmer ground when attempting to predict a second episode in someone who has already had a first episode, and subsequent episodes in those who have had more than one episode. However, there are a number of factors, some patient-related and others environmental, that conspire to worsen the clinical state. Some factors can be transient, such as life events, which may lead to decompensation and possibly spontaneous return to baseline with the passing of the disturbing life event. Relapse can be precipitated by a single factor, but is often the result of the snowballing effect of multiple insults, which are shown in Figure 15.1.

Factors associated with RELAPSE are:

- **Relapse history** predicts subsequent relapses
- **Expressed emotion** (criticism or over involvement), particularly by family members, predisposes to relapse
- **Life events**, both positive and negative, commonly precede relapse. Breakdown in relationships, being evicted from home, loss of a job, poor grades in school are some examples
- **Alcohol and substance abuse** is a very common reason for relapse
- **Physical illnesses** that are concomitant, such as infections, new head injury, seizures, or nutritional impairment can lead to worsening of symptoms

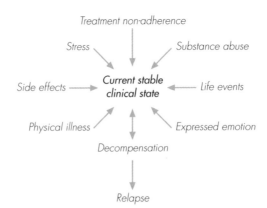

Figure 15.1 Decompensation and relapse risk factors.

- **Stopping medications** is by far the most common reason for relapse
- **Emergent side effects** such as akathisia, which used to be quite a common reason for relapse, fortunately decreased with the advent of atypical antipsychotic drugs (APDs).

Discussing these predictors of relapse candidly with a patient, particularly with the first episode of psychosis, can go a long way in preventing relapse. Simplified further, patients and their families should be informed of the Three S's – **Stress**, **Substance abuse** and **Stopping medications** – which are key reasons for relapse.

It is also important to develop, with the assistance of the patient and family, a list of early **warning symptoms** that are harbingers of relapse. Each patient will have unique path to decompensation or relapse. For one patient the early warning sign may be the emergence of sleep difficulty, while in another patient it may be the return of auditory hallucinations.

Management of decompensation

The challenge in managing decompensation is deciding when to take a stance of watchful inaction versus active intervention, because mild worsening of clinical state can simply be normal variation in response to life's vicissitudes, and the patient returns to the previous better state relatively quickly. Acting too quickly and aggressively can be demoralizing to the patient; it engenders a feeling that they are completely at the mercy of the healthcare system with no capability to manage the illness on their own. On the other hand, when the rate of decompensation is rapid it is best to act quickly.

In patients having multiple relapses, the 'march' of clinical worsening towards relapse tends to be the same from one episode to the next. Thus, knowing well the psychiatric history of the patient can go a long way towards helping decide when and how to respond to change in clinical state. Also, a good therapeutic relationship with the patient and family is critical to successful relapse-prevention interventions.

Measures that can reverse decompensation include:
- supportive therapy for general support
- case management to assist with living; situations that may be stressful
- psychoeducation to reinforce the goals of treatment

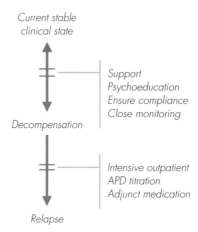

Figure 15.2 Interventions aimed at reversing decompensation and preventing relapse.

- ensuring treatment adherence because clinical worsening can be both a consequence and a cause of treatment non-adherence (Figure 15.2).

If decompensation is clearly heading towards a relapse, then initiate:

- intensive outpatient program (partial hospital)
- medication titration
- adjunctive medication (e.g. benzodiazepines)
- hospitalization, if required.

Management of relapse

The management of relapse is the management of an acute episode. The steps taken to prevent a full-blown relapse may be helpful in mitigating the severity and duration of the relapse. Because each episode of relapse is more difficult to treat than the previous episode, it is worthwhile to spend considerable effort in preventing relapses. With each relapse comes the responsibility of devising an even better program of relapse prevention for the patient.

Relapse prevention

After the first episode of psychosis, the task of treatment is to keep the patient well for as long as possible. Thus, preventing relapses is the goal of maintenance treatment. Everything we have discussed about treatment so far is applicable to relapse prevention. However, it helps to frame these treatments as a formal program (give it a name); it helps keep the focus on active prevention of relapse, not just treatment as usual.

Educating the patient and family about early signs and symptoms associated with relapse goes a long way towards relapse prevention. As noted above, each patient will have a unique pattern of relapse that tends to be the same for each episode. Table 15.1 contains a very comprehensive listing of early warning signs, developed by Birchwood and colleagues (1989).

Summary

- The course of schizophrenic illness for many patients involves episodes of decompensation (transitory clinical worsening) and relapse (clinical worsening that requires active intervention). The goal of maintenance treatment is to minimize the frequency and severity of relapse.
- Each episode of relapse becomes harder to treat than the previous one.
- A variety of factors are predictive of relapse and increase its risk: **relapse history, expressed emotion, life events, alcohol and substance abuse, physical illnesses, stopping medications,** and **emergent side effects.** Discuss these predictors with patients and families at the beginning of treatment.
- Identify early warning symptoms that are unique to given patient.
- Management of decompensation involves taking a stance of watchful inaction in the case of mild worsening of clinical state. Act quickly when the rate of decompensation is rapid. Knowing well a patient's psychiatric history can help decide when and how to respond to change in clinical state. Give appropriate supportive therapy, apply case management, psychoeducation, and encourage treatment adherence.
- A good therapeutic relationship with the patient and family is critical to successful relapse prevention interventions.
- Relapse prevention involves an intensive outpatient program, medication titration, adjunctive medication, and possible hospitalization.
- Relapse management is the same as management of an acute episode.

Table 15.1 Early warning signs of impending relapse

Thinking and perception	Feelings	Behaviors
Thoughts are racing	Feeling helpless or useless	Difficulty sleeping
Senses seem sharper	Feeling afraid of going crazy	Speech comes out jumbled, filled with odd words
Thinking you have special powers	Feeling sad or low	Talking or smiling to yourself
Thinking that you can read other people's minds	Feeling anxious and restless	Acting suspiciously as if being watched
Thinking that other people can read your mind	Feeling increasingly religious	Behaving oddly for no reason
Receiving personal messages from the TV or radio	Feeling like you're being watched	Spending time alone
Having difficulty making decisions	Feeling isolated	Neglecting your appearance
Experiencing strange sensations	Feeling tired or lacking energy	Acting like you are somebody else
Preoccupied about one or two things	Feeling confused or puzzled	Not seeing people
Thinking you might be somebody else	Feeling forgetful or far away	Not eating
Seeing visions or things others cannot see	Feeling in another world	Not leaving the house
Thinking people are talking about you	Feeling strong and powerful	Behaving like a child
Thinking people are against you	Feeling unable to cope with everyday tasks	Refusing to do simple requests
Having more nightmares	Feeling like you are being punished	Drinking more
Having difficulty concentrating	Feeling like you cannot trust other people	Smoking more
Thinking bizarre things	Feeling irritable	Movements are slow
Thinking your thoughts are controlled	Feeling like you do not need sleep	Unable to sit down for long
Hearing voices	Feeling guilty	Behaving aggressively
Thinking that a part of you has changed shape		

Source: Birchwood M, Smith J, Macmillan F, *et al.* (1989): Predicting relapse in schizophrenia: the development and implementation of an early signs monitoring system using patients and families as observers, a preliminary investigation. *Psychol Med* 19: 649–56.

chapter 16

Suicide and violence

You ever-gentle gods, take my breath from me;
Let not my worser spirit tempt me again
To die before you please. King Lear, William Shakespeare (1564–1616)

Suicide

Schizophrenia is a disorder with quite high mortality. About half of all patients with schizophrenia attempt suicide and 10–13% of patients die from suicide. In spite of advances in treatment over the last half-century, the rates of suicide and parasuicide (suicide attempts) have not declined; in fact, they have risen according to some research. Thus, suicide assessment and prevention becomes an important component in the treatment of schizophrenia.

Risk factors
A variety of risk factors are associated with suicide in general and schizophrenia in particular, which do not necessarily overlap. For example, being male is a risk factor for suicide in the general population but it is a less robust predictor of suicide in the case of schizophrenia. Predictors of suicide in schizophrenia include high premorbid IQ and good premorbid achievement predisposing to failed expectations, and early relapse or disability leading to a fear of mental deterioration; psychological factors include hopelessness, perceived loss of control over the illness, and experience of stigma. Low levels of suicidal ideation early in the illness may be predictive of subsequent suicidal behavior, independent of depression. The following are

established risk factors for schizophrenia (SADHEART).

Suicide risk in schizophrenia is greatest 'early' on:

Single
Alcohol and substance abuse
Depressed mood
Hopelessness
Early phase of illness
Achieving highly premorbidly
Revolving door admissions
Treatment failure

- Earlier (i.e. younger) age
- Early age at onset of illness
- Early phase of illness
- Early after recovery from first episode of illness
- Early after discharge; risk of completed suicide is highest in the immediate post-discharge period
- Early low-level suicide ideation may predict later suicidality

The clinician should be vigilant for subtle and early indications of suicidality, monitor such patients closely, and institute appropriate interventions.

Violence

From portrayals in the media, one would conclude that patients with schizophrenia routinely indulge in violent behavior. In fact, there are little convincing data that aggressive or homicidal behavior is more common in persons with this illness than in the general population. Aggression is an accompaniment of irritability, loss of impulse control, and neurological dysfunction, and is seen in many neurological and psychiatric disorders. However, the enduring image that patients with schizophrenia are prone to unpredictable violence has done a great disservice to them. However, some patients do indulge in aggressive behavior, often as a result of bizarre hallucinations or delusions.

It is useful to consider violence as either transient or persistent because such a classification has management implications.

Transient violence occurs in the context of excitation and hyperarousal, usually in the midst of an acute episode of psychosis, particularly when leading up to or during hospitalization. Once the episode of psychosis is treated, the violence recedes and there is generally no continued aggressive behavior as long as treatment is continued and effective.

Persistent violence is committed by a very small proportion of patients with schizophrenia. Unlike transiently violent patients, these patients remain at high risk for violent behavior, even when receiving adequate treatment and not in hyperarousal state.

Risk factors for violent behavior (predicting DANGER) are:
Delusions
Antisocial traits
Neurologic impairment
Gender – male
Ethanol and drug use
Repeated violence

Management of violence

Violence is a medical emergency. The first order of business is physical safety of all the parties. This may involve some form of restraint, but only as last resort. A quick, but careful, assessment should be performed to determine contributors to violence, particularly medical conditions. With a working diagnosis in hand, appropriate interventions can be instituted, which may include parenteral benzodiazepines (such as lorazepam) or antipsychotic drugs (APDs) such as droperidol or haloperidol.

Once the violence has abated and treatment is well underway, the episode(s) of violence should be reviewed to determine whether it was transient or persistent in nature. If transient, then no specific violence management may be required other than ensuring continued treatment. On the other hand, if the violence appears to be enduring, review of current pharmacological treatment and enrollment into a violence prevention program is necessary. Atypical APDs, particularly clozapine, have been found to reduce violent behavior. Violence reduction programs vary considerably, but most have the following components:

- cueing (identify signs of anger)
- cognitive behavior therapy
- cognitive remediation
- anger management
- coping skills
- relaxation techniques
- structured environment
- leisure activities.

Summary

- Half of all patients with schizophrenia attempt suicide and at least 10% of patients die from suicide.
- A variety of risk factors are associated with suicide in schizophrenia: single status, alcohol and substance abuse, depressed mood, hopelessness, early phase of illness, achieving highly premorbidly, revolving door admissions, and treatment failure.
- Suicide risk in schizophrenia is greatest early in the course of illness, at a younger age, during the pot-discharge period, and associated with low-level suicidal ideation.
- With regard to violence, patients with schizophrenia are in general no more aggressive than the general population.
- Aggression is an accompaniment of irritability, loss of impulse control, and neurological dysfunction.
- Violence can be **transient** or **persistent**. Transient violence is seen with excitation and hyperarousal, and with treatment it is controlled. Persistent violence is committed by a very small proportion of patients with schizophrenia; it can occur even when receiving adequate treatment and not in hyperarousal state.
- A variety of risk factors are predictive of violence. One of the most robust predictor is previous history of violence. Others include persecutory delusions, lack of insight, substance abuse, treatment non-adherence; neurologic impairment and antisocial traits are associated with persistent violence, and male gender predisposes.
- Violence is a medical emergency and management includes: seeing to the physical safety of all the parties; quick, but careful, assessment; pharmacological interventions (benzodiazepines, droperidol, or haloperidol).
- Persistent violence requires referral to violence reduction programs.

chapter 17

Achieving recovery

My head's sore no more
No one's showing me the door
Ma, see, I tiptoed past that mine
And now, just maybe, I'll be fine

All the information in the preceding chapters lays the foundation for helping patients achieve recovery. What constitutes *recovery* is still not agreed upon universally. Some define it as the absence of major symptoms without taking into account the level of psychosocial functioning. Others define recovery as complete absence of symptoms with no further requirement for treatment and no longer viewing the patient as psychiatrically ill. Obviously, rates of recovery depend on which criteria are utilized.

Having very modest aims for recovery (e.g. absence of positive symptoms as the only criterion) can blunt outcome, because all that can be done for the patient may not have been considered. On the other hand, too lofty recovery goals that are not achieved can lead to demoralization. The most sensible approach is an individualized one, since no 'one-size-fits-all' criteria can be applied to all patients. For each patient there are unique interacting factors that influence the extent of recovery (Figure 17.1). These may be categorized as **patient-related** (e.g. substance abuse), **environmental** (e.g. family interaction), **treatment-related** (e.g. appropriate antipsychotic drug [APD] dose) and **biological** factors (age at onset of illness).

Recent research indicates that the following ten factors are important for achieving recovery:

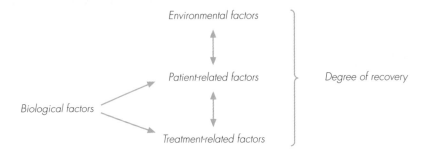

Figure 17.1 Relations between factors influencing recovery.

Access to care. Continuous treatment and multimodal approaches (APDs, individual and group therapy, rehabilitation) are critical to achieving recovery.

Cognitive abilities. Adequate cognitive skills (working memory, perception skills and problem-solving abilities) are predictive of recovery.

Duration of untreated psychosis. Delay in treatment of the initial episode is associated with greater difficulty in achieving remission, and can negatively impact long-term outcome.

Family relationships. Family emotional support decreases relapse rate, while family stress increases the risk for relapse.

Initial response to medication. The rapidity of treatment response is a predictor of good outcome. Most patients with successful outcome report good response to the first APD used.

Personal history. Later age at onset of illness and good premorbid functioning are associated with recovery. Patients who have good outcome tend to have a higher IQ, a college degree, and good work history.

Substance abuse. Almost half of the patients abuse substances (see below), which is associated with relapse and poorer outcome.

Social skills. No more than mild deficits in social skills are associated with favorable outcome.

Supportive therapy. Almost all patients who recover report being in regular therapy and having positive relations with clinical team members.

Treatment adherence. As has mentioned throughout the book, non-adherence does not bode well for short-term remission and long-term recovery.

Co-morbid conditions

A variety of conditions are commonly observed along with (co-morbid) schizophrenia that significantly impact on treatment and outcome, and ultimately recovery. Thus, there should be heightened awareness of these conditions when assessing and treating schizophrenia.

Depression

Depressive symptoms are common in schizophrenia, and may be part of the prodrome, the florid phase, or follow the first episode (postpsychotic depression). Depression occurs in 25–40% of patients, and is associated with increased suicidality and poor outcome.

The relationship between depression and schizophrenia has not been fully elucidated. Depression in schizophrenia may be due to the appearance of insight about the nature of illness and its lifetime implications. It may be integral to the schizophrenic illness, or reflect another disorder such as schizoaffective disorder or major depression co-occurring with schizophrenia. First-episode patients tend to have more severe depression compared with multi-episode patients. Persistent hopelessness at discharge is associated with poor outcome a year later.

Depressive symptoms seen in patients with schizophrenia present a diagnostic challenge. Depression accompanying psychosis is seen in major depression and the depressive phase of bipolar disorder. Neuroleptic-induced parkinsonism and primary negative symptoms can be mistaken for depression.

Co-morbid depression must be treated promptly. Selective serotonin reuptake inhibitors (SSRIs) are quite effective in treating depression in schizophrenia, unlike the older antidepressants. In the case of antidepressant-resistant depression, atypical APDs, particularly clozapine, have been helpful – more so than typical APDs.

Substance abuse

Substance abuse is very common in patients with schizophrenia; as many as half of all patients will abuse substances during their lifetime. The most common are nicotine and alcohol, followed by cannabis and cocaine. Dual diagnosis (substance abuse + schizophrenia) is more common in young males with lower education. Family history of substance abuse and conduct disorders further increase the risk for substance abuse.

Substance abuse can precede, accompany, or follow the first psychotic episode. The physiological effects of abused substances tend to occur at much lower quantities in patients with schizophrenia. The course of substance abuse in schizophrenia tends to be chronic with multiple relapses. Substance abuse has many dire consequences, including:

- higher relapse rates
- treatment non-adherence
- blunting APD effectiveness
- violence
- depression
- suicide
- increased risk of injury and medical illness
- financial problems
- legal problems
- housing problems
- increased use of emergency services.

Achieving abstinence is not easy and requires an integrated approach to assessment and treatment. The most important component of assessment is screening for substance abuse. This includes asking patients directly about substance abuse, urine drug screening, and collateral sources of information. Treatment consists of psychoeducation, enhancing motivation to quit (motivational interviewing), psychological interventions (e.g. cognitive behavior therapy), and pharmacological approaches (e.g. clozapine).

Smoking

Cigarette smoking by patients with schizophrenia exceeds the rates in the general US population by two- to threefold. The prevalence of cigarette smoking in patients with schizophrenia is between 70% and 90%, compared to 35–55% for all other psychiatric patients and 30–35% for the general population. It is not entirely clear why patients with schizophrenia smoke at such high rates. Reasons suggested include a genetic basis, a method of self-treatment, or an underlying neurobiological cause (nicotinergic deficit). Many patients start smoking after the first episode of psychosis. The nature of smoking seems to differ as well (smoking high-tar cigarettes and for longer periods, inhaling more deeply).

Smoking offsets the sedative effects from psychotropic medications. It has been shown that smoking lowers blood levels of many psychoactive agents, including APDs, by activating hepatic enzyme systems thereby increasing their metabolism, and may help overcome akathisia, dystonia, and parkinsonism. These findings lend support to the idea of self-medication – more correctly, self-treatment of side effects. Thus, medication dosing has to be adjusted to smoking status, and in the event of sudden smoking cessation the blood levels of drugs can rise dramatically resulting in toxicity. Dose reduction is often required in such situations.

Regardless of the reasons for high rates of smoking, it is associated with significant medical morbidity except, ironically, lower rates of lung cancer. Patients should be referred to smoking cessation programs, and coordinate closely with psychiatric care. Pharmacological aids to smoking cessation include nicotine patches and gum, bupropion, and possibly clozapine.

Summary

- What constitutes *recovery* is still not agreed upon universally. Some define it as the absence of major symptoms without taking into account the level of psychosocial functioning. Others define recovery as complete absence of symptoms with no further requirement for treatment and no longer viewing the patient as psychiatrically ill.
- Recovery assessment and treatment planning should be individualized. Each patient has a unique set of interacting factors that influence the extent of recovery.
- There are at least ten factors important for achieving recovery: **access to care; cognitive abilities; duration of untreated psychosis; family relationships; initial response to medication; personal history; substance abuse; social skills; supportive therapy; and treatment adherence.**
- Co-morbidity can significantly impact treatment and outcome. **Depressive symptoms** are common in schizophrenia, occurring in 25–40% of patients. First-episode patients tend to have more severe depression

compared with multi-episode patients. Persistent hopelessness at discharge is associated with poor outcome. Depression accompanying psychosis is seen in major depression, bipolar disorder, and parkinsonism, and primary negative symptoms can be mistaken for depression. SSRIs, and some atypical APDs, are quite effective in treating depression in schizophrenia.

- As many as half of all patients with schizophrenia will **abuse substances** during their lifetime; the most common are nicotine and alcohol, followed by cannabis and cocaine. Substance abuse has many dire consequences and treatment is not easy. An integrated approach to assessment and treatment is required. Treatment consists of psychoeducation, motivational interviewing, cognitive behavior therapy and pharmacotherapy.

- Patients with schizophrenia have the highest rates of cigarette smoking (70%–90%). Patients tend to smoke high-tar cigarettes and inhale more deeply. Smoking counters the sedative effects from psychotropic medications, lowers blood levels of many psychoactive agents, and may help overcome extrapyramidal side effects. Smoking is associated with significant medical morbidity and patients should be referred to smoking cessation programs. Pharmacological aids against smoking include nicotine patches and gum, bupropion, and possibly clozapine.

chapter 18

History of schizophrenia

Only the man who is familiar with the art and science of the past is competent to aid its progress in the future.

Christian Albert Theodor Billroth (1829–1894)

Texts from Egypt and Mesopotamia from the 2nd millennium BC, as well as the *Atharvaveda*, an ancient Indian scripture (ca. 1000 BC), contain descriptions of mental derangement. However, descriptions consistent with the modern conception of schizophrenia show up only in the 18th century. Some psychiatric historians suggest that schizophrenia is an ancient disorder, while others argue that it is a relatively modern one, not more than two centuries old. This is more than an academic debate. If schizophrenia is indeed of recent origin (recency hypothesis), then it suggests that historically recent changes, likely environmental, may be responsible for the emergence of schizophrenia.

The history of schizophrenia is the history of keen clinical observation. Psychiatrists had the opportunity to observe the natural progression of schizophrenia over the course of years, if not entire lifetimes of patients. This allowed careful descriptions of clinical syndromes and their natural courses. Nosology was in vogue during the 19th century, leading to a variety of systems of classification of mental disorders. Below is a glimpse at a few of the luminaries who have brought the concept of schizophrenia thus far.

John Haslam (1764–1844)

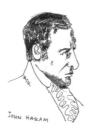

JOHN HASLAM

In 1810, Haslam published a book titled, *Illustrations of Madness: Exhibiting a Singular Case of Insanity, And a No Less Remarkable Difference in Medical Opinions: Developing the Nature of An Assailment, And the Manner of Working Events; with a Description of Tortures Experienced by Bomb-Bursting, Lobster-Cracking and Lengthening the Brain. Embellished with a Curious Plate.* The book contains a detailed description of James Tilly Matthews' psychosis, the first clear description of schizophrenia.

Phillipe Pinel (1745–1826)

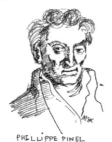

PHILLIPPE PINEL

Pinel's dictum to his students, still valid today: 'Take written notes at the sickbed and record the entire course of severe illness'. He is considered one of the founders of psychiatry. His 'Moral Treatment' was the first attempt at individual psychotherapy. He emphasized hygiene, physical exercise, and work for his patients.

Benedict Morel (1809–1873)

In 1860, Morel introduced the term *dementia praecoce* to refer to a mental deterioration 'for an illness beginning in adolescence and leading to gradual deterioration'.

Karl Kahlbaum (1828–1899)

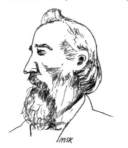

CARL KAHLBAUM

Kahlbaum was the director of his own institution for the mentally ill in Görlitz, Germany. He was the first to distinguish between the clinical pictures and the diseases in which they occur. He coined the term *Katatonia* in 1868.

Ewald Hecker (1843–1909)

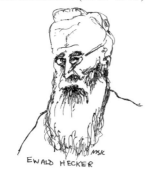

EWALD HECKER

Emil Kraepelin (1856–1926)

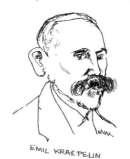

EMIL KRAEPELIN

Eugen Bleuler (1857–1939)

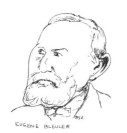

EUGENE BLEULER

Hecker worked with Kahlbaum in Görlitz, after which he bought his own psychiatric hospital in Wiesbaden, Germany. He was never given an academic position because of his liberal views. His classic paper on *hebephrenia* was published in 1871, in which is described a syndrome of early-onset psychosis with a deteriorating course, with 'silly' affect, behavioral oddities, and thought disorder.

Undoubtedly one of the most important figures in psychiatry. In 1883, Kraepelin wrote his *Compendium der Psychiatrie*. In its sixth edition (1899) he presented the distinction between manic–depressive psychosis and dementia praecox. Kraepelin also distinguished at least three clinical varieties of dementia praecox: catatonia, hebephrenia, and paranoia. Kraepelin campaigned against smoking and alcohol. In the Munich psychiatric clinic all alcohol was banned and patients were offered lemonade (*Kraepelinsekt*).

Bleuler coined the term 'schizophrenia' to describe a 'splitting' of mental functions. He wrote thus:

> 'I call dementia praecox "schizophrenia" because (as I hope to demonstrate) the "splitting" of the different psychic functions is one of its most important characteristics. For the sake of convenience, I use the word in the singular although it is apparent that the group includes several diseases.'

He emphasized that certain symptoms,

(Bleuler's four 'As': autism, ambivalence, disturbances in association, and affectivity), were 'fundamental' while other symptoms, such as delusions and hallucinations – 'accessory symptoms' – because they were found in other disorders.

Kurt Schneider (1887–1967)

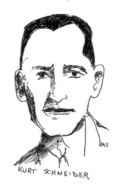

KURT SCHNEIDER

Schneider identified certain types of delusions and hallucinations as being characteristic of schizophrenia ('First Rank Symptoms'). These criteria, published in 1959, represented a narrow concept of schizophrenia, which was more popular in European psychiatry.

Adolf Meyer (1866–1950)

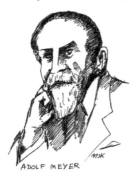

ADOLF MEYER

Meyer is rightly known as 'the dean of American psychiatry'. He advocated a thorough understanding of the patient as a whole person. He also argued for integrating psychology and biology into a single system, psychobiology, which was to be applied to assessment and treatment, with the goal of helping the patient adjust to life and change. A component of the therapy, called 'habit training', was to help patients, including those with schizophrenia, to modify unhealthy adjustments by guidance, suggestion, and re-education. He considered schizophrenia being caused by harmful habits in conjunction with biological factors as well as heredity.

Sigmund Freud (1856–1939)

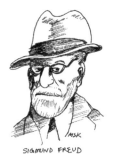

SIGMUND FREUD

Freud's contributions towards understanding schizophrenia include the concepts of projection and primary narcissism. Projection is a defense mechanism, operating unconsciously, in which emotionally unacceptable impulses are rejected and attributed to others. He referred to schizophrenia as 'paraphrenia', and was doubtful that psychoanalysis could help.

In spite of the progress made during the previous century, the early and mid-20th century was marked by descriptive and diagnostic inconsistency. Further, the lack of understanding of etiopathology of the illness contributed to significant variations in the frequency of diagnosis of schizophrenia during. During the 1960s the World Health Organization (WHO) took the initiative to establish a set of criteria which gradually evolved towards the International Classification of Diseases. A multinational study, conducted by the WHO, using standardized criteria, revealed similar worldwide prevalence of schizophrenia. Currently, there are several (at least 15) competing criteria and there is no general agreement as to which is the best. The latest diagnostic scheme, Diagnostic and Statistical Manual, Fourth Edition (DSM-IV, American Psychiatric Association 1994), has incorporated several significant changes in the diagnostic criteria for schizophrenia. Although there are critiques of the validity of these diagnostic criteria, the ICD and DSM have improved diagnostic reliability and understanding of schizophrenia. Further refinements in diagnosis will likely come from advancements in genetics and neurobiology.

Summary

The history of mental illness extends back over 3000 years, recorded in early writings from Egypt, Mesopotamia and India.

Descriptions of schizophrenia, as defined today, appear in the 18th century. The earliest best description was provided by John Haslam in 1810.

Schizophrenia may be a relatively modern disorder (*recency hypothesis*), some have argued, suggesting that the effects of modernity, probably environmental, may be responsible for the emergence of schizophrenia.

The history of the concept of schizophrenia is the history of keen clinical observation and classification by psychiatrists during the 19th and 20th centuries (Table 18.1).

Table 18.1 Important contributions to the concept of schizophrenia

Phillipe Pinel (1745–1826)	Invented *Moral Treatment*
Benedict Morel (1809–1873)	Introduced the term *dementia praecoce*
Karl Kahlbaum (1828–1899)	He coined the term *Katatonia*
Ewald Hecker (1843–1909)	He gave us *hebephrenia*
Emil Kraepelin (1856–1926)	He presented the distinction between *dementia praecox* and manic-depressive psychosis
Eugen Bleuler (1857–1939)	Bleuler coined the term *schizophrenia* Bleuler's four 'As' (autism, ambivalence, disturbances in association, and affectivity)
Kurt Schneider (1887–1967)	Defined the *first rank symptoms*
Adolf Meyer (1866–1950)	He considered schizophrenia was caused by harmful habits in conjunction with biological factors as well as heredity.
Sigmund Freud (1856–1939)	Introduced concepts of *projection* and primary narcissism.

Recent advances in the concept of schizophrenia have included the application of formal diagnostic criteria, based by research findings and expert consensus. The following are the most widely used:

- International Classification of Diseases (currently, 10th edition – ICD-10)
- Diagnostic and Statistical Manual of Mental Disorders (currently Fourth Edition, Text Revision–DSM-IV-TR)

Further refinements in diagnosis will likely come from advancements in genetics and neurobiology.

chapter 19

Who gets schizophrenia and why?

The apple never falls far from the tree!
So how come blame me
When it's just egg and sperm off key

In discussing who might develop schizophrenia and why that might be the case, there are genetic and epigenetic factors to consider. Since the precise pathology of schizophrenia is not known, epidemiological methods (Greek *epi* = upon; *demos* = people; *logos* = word, discourse; the study of occurrence of diseases in human populations) are used to investigate the possible determinants of schizophrenia.

Incidence is the number of newly diagnosed cases during a specific time period. In any given year, 3 to 6 individuals will be newly diagnosed with schizophrenia out of a population of 10 000 (incidence rate: 0.3–0.6/1000).

Prevalence is the number of cases of a disease that are present in a particular population at a given time (*point prevalence*). Current research indicates a prevalence of 4–7/1000 persons. There are approximately 50 million individuals worldwide diagnosed with schizophrenia, including 2.2 million in the USA, 250 000 in Great Britain, 8.7 million in India, 12 million in China, 280 000 people in Canada, and 285 000 in Australia.

> **Lifetime prevalence** is the number of individuals in the population who will develop the disorder at some point during their lifetime. Latest research indicates that the lifetime prevalence of schizophrenia is approximately 0.5%, lower than the traditionally quoted 1%.

There are **geographical variations** in prevalence rates, both higher and lower than the worldwide average. Regions of higher prevalence (also called geographical isolates) include Croatia, some islands in Micronesia, northern Sweden and Finland, and parts of Ireland. Lower prevalence is seen in Botswana, Ghana, Papua New Guinea, and Taiwan.

There are also **communities** with prevalence rates higher than the region in which they are located – examples are aboriginals of Australia and natives of northern Canada. Jamaican immigrants in the UK, compared with Jamaicans in Jamaica, appear to have a higher rate of schizophrenia, which does not appear to be due to stress. Lower prevalence rates are seen in the Amish and Hutterite communities in the USA.

Is schizophrenia familial?

Eugen Bleuler had noted that relatives of patients with schizophrenia were often 'tainted by hereditary mental disease'. In recent years, the genetic basis of this illness has been well established, to the extent that Seymour Kety said, 'If schizophrenia is a myth, it is a genetically transmitted myth!' It is well established that schizophrenia aggregates in families. The reason for this could be either a shared family environment (*nurture*) or due to genes (*nature*) or a combination (*gene–environment interaction*).

Family, twin, and adoption studies have demonstrated that the chance of developing schizophrenia increases with biological proximity to the affected individual, establishing that *heritability* is a major risk factor. The risk of developing schizophrenia increases from about 0.5% in the general population to almost 50% if both parents are affected, or if an identical twin is affected, with various risk estimates in between depending on degree of relatedness (Figure 19.1). Based on these findings, heritability has been estimated at 70%, which is the proportion of liability variance in the population that is accounted for by genetic factors. Thus, 30% of the variance is not accounted for by genetic transmission and has to be accounted for by non-genetic factors.

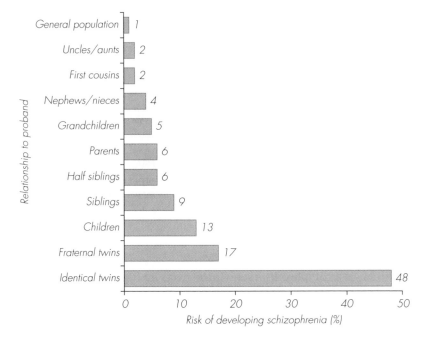

Figure 19.1 Risk of developing schizophrenia as affected by closeness of relatives with the disease (from Gottesman, 1991).

How is schizophrenia transmitted?

The specific mode of transmission of schizophrenia is unclear, but several models have been proposed (Table 19.1).

Evidence to date is incompatible with either a single major locus model or a simple polygenic model; a more complex multifactorial/threshold model and a major gene against a polygenic/multifactorial background remain as possibilities. Progress in clarifying this issue has been limited because of unclear clinical boundaries of schizophrenia, the likely involvement of multiple genes, each with small effect, and genetic heterogeneity. Further there is the possibility of major environmental and developmental, and epigenetic determinants that influence the eventual development of schizophrenia.

Table 19.1 Models of genetic transmission

Distinct heterogeneity model	Schizophrenia is a collection of several diseases; each associated with single major locus (SML), and inherited dominantly or recessively. In addition, there are sporadic cases
Monogenic models (single major locus models)	Schizophrenia might be a single-gene disorder with variable expression or reduced penetrance (probability of manifesting a trait given a particular genotype)
Multifactorial-polygenic threshold model	Schizophrenia results from (small) effects of multiple genes interacting with a variety of environmental factors
A mixed or combined model	The model includes the elements of some, or all, of the above

What is transmitted?

Schizophrenia is a complex disorder which affects multiple domains of functioning, which *per se* cannot be transmitted via genes. Rather, what may be transmitted is a *liability* for developing the illness. This liability may express itself as poor psychosocial functioning, oddness, or non-affective psychoses. Biological relatives of schizophrenic probands (Latin *probandus*; the one to be tested) have a higher prevalence of schizophrenia and schizotypal personality disorder; these disorders have been considered to represent **schizophrenia spectrum disorders**. However, general behavioral disturbances, such as 'oddness', are rather crude indicators of risk.

Endophenotypes (illness traits that are between the phenotype and genotype), such as SPEM (Smooth Pursuit Eye Movement) dysfunction and sustained attentional deficits (Figure 19.2), may be more refined indicators of risk and serve as biological **vulnerability markers**, and are increasingly being utilized as a research strategy in genetic studies.

The search for schizophrenia genes

Advances in molecular genetic techniques and the recent mapping of the human genome have raised the hope for identifying specific genes and to resolve genetic heterogeneity in schizophrenia. The final objective of gene-hunting is to identify gene products which will lead to working out the pathophysiology of schizophrenia and ultimately its cure (Figure 19.3).

There have been some advances in identifying genes for schizophrenia utilizing association studies, which measure the relative frequency of a particular polymorphism associated with the trait of interest in a population (Table 19.2).

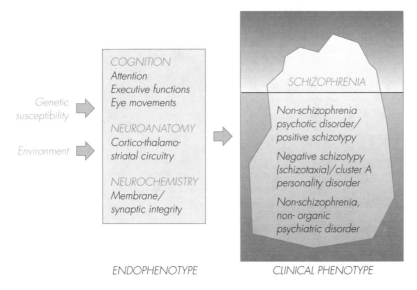

Figure 19.2 Endophenotypes are intermediate to gene/environment risk and the phenotype.

Environmental factors

As noted above, genes have a prominent, but not exclusive role in the pathogenesis of schizophrenia. There are several biological environmental factors that consistently have been found to be associated with schizophrenia (Table 19.3), although their pathogenic mechanism has not been deciphered.

Gene–environment interaction

It is likely that genetic and biologic vulnerability underlying schizophrenia makes an individual more vulnerable to stress. Thus, the illness results from an interaction between stress and vulnerability, a model originally proposed by Joseph Zubin (1900–1990). In such a model, it is postulated that there is an enduring and variable degree of biological (likely genetic) vulnerability to developing the clinical syndrome. Interacting with this vulnerability is internal and external stress that transforms vulnerability into the clinical syndrome. There exists a hypothetical *inverse* relationship between the degree of vulnerability and the degree of stress required for emergence of schizophrenic illness. Thus, the greater the genetic load the less psychosocial stress needed to trigger the illness (see Figure 19.4).

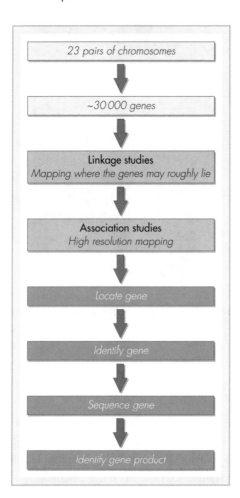

Figure 19.3 A simplified pathway to uncovering the schizophrenia genes.

Table 19.2 Genes of interest in schizophrenia and their loci

Gene product (gene)	Locus
Dysbindin (*DTNBP1*)	6p22.3
Neuregulin 1 (*NRG1*)	8p12–p21
Catechol-O-methyltransferase (*COMT*)	22q11
Regulator of G-protein signaling-4 (*RGS4*)	1q21–22

Table 19.3 Environmental risk factors

Perinatal complications	History of pregnancy and birth complications (e.g. pre-eclampsia, prematurity, low birth weight) are present in about 25% of patients, more often in males. Hypoxic brain injury may be one mechanism mediating the effects of birth complications. Prenatal exposure to influenza in the 2nd trimester and nutritional deficiencies are other environmental factors that increase the risk of schizophrenia
Season of birth	In the northern hemisphere, schizophrenia patients tend to be born more frequently between January and April; in the southern hemisphere, the same is true between July and September. It has been suggested that viral infections may account for this
Minor physical anomalies	These are minor structural deviations found in the head, eyes, mouth, ears, hands and feet. These include wide-set eyes, high palate in the mouth, adherent ear lobes, abnormal hair whorls, and abnormal dermatoglyphics. These anomalies are 'archeological' evidence of maldevelopment occurring at the same time as major brain development (i.e. the 1st and perhaps early 2nd trimesters of pregnancy)
Cannabis abuse	There is increasing evidence that heavy cannabis abuse during adolescence increases the risk for later schizophrenia. It is not clear whether cannabis abuse causes schizophrenia or precipitates the illness

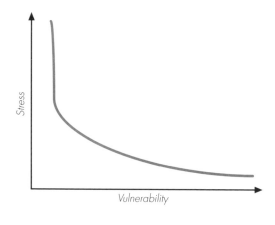

Figure 19.4 Relations between stress and vulnerability in the development of schizophrenia.

chapter 20

Neurobiology of schizophrenia

Inside, out
What am I about?
Cut me, poke me, view my brain
Call me, tell me, sane or insane?

Schizophrenia has stubbornly resisted yielding its secrets, despite a century of research. That said, however, much has been learned about disturbances in the brain *associated* with the disorder. Recent studies utilizing neuroimaging, neurophysiology, neurochemistry, and neuropathological methods have advanced our understanding of brain circuitry and biochemical underpinnings of the pathophysiology of schizophrenia.

Early studies largely relied on postmortem examination of the brains of mostly older patients with chronic schizophrenia or brain scans in patients with established schizophrenia, many of whom were treated with medications. It was difficult, therefore, to tease apart the effects of the illness from those of aging, illness chronicity, and medications. Studies of individuals in the early phases of schizophrenia, especially those in the first episode, have recently advanced our understanding considerably.

Neuroanatomical alterations

Over a quarter-century ago, computed tomography (CT) showed that patients with schizophrenia have a reduction in brain tissue as evidenced by enlarged cerebral ventricles (Figure 20.1). Several magnetic resonance imaging (MRI) studies have confirmed significant abnormalities in brain

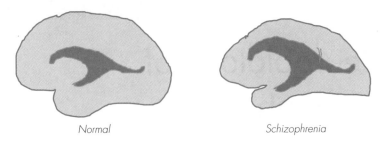

Normal   *Schizophrenia*

Figure 20.1 Ventriculomegaly and cortical atrophy.

structure in patients with schizophrenia and have firmly established that schizophrenia is indeed a brain disease.

It had been known from the early part of the 20th century that schizophrenic patients might frequently show enlargement of the cerebral ventricles, as shown in pneumoencephalographic studies. The advent of CT scanning in the 1970s confirmed the observations that lateral ventricles are enlarged in a substantial proportion of schizophrenic patients; these data were replicated with subsequent MRI studies (Figure 20.2).

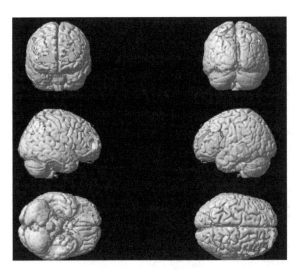

Figure 20.2 Structural brain abnormalities in schizophrenia. Brain regions with gray matter volume reductions are shown as shaded areas.

MRI research has delineated the following structural brain abnormalities:

- reduced brain volume of about 5–10%, especially with reductions in gray matter;
- enlarged lateral and third ventricles;
- decreased volume of the superior temporal gyri and medial temporal cortex, notably the hippocampus and amygdale;
- subtle reductions in the volume of the prefrontal cortex;
- reductions in subcortical structures such as cerebellar, caudate, and thalamic volumes;
- reductions in the size of the corpus callosum;
- reversal or loss of the asymmetry of the cerebral hemispheres.

Neuroanatomical alterations appear to be present at the onset of the illness. Whether these abnormalities are **static or progressive** has been an important question. Static 'lesions' would suggest that the pathological 'event' has already occurred in the past and thus may not be reversible. On the other hand, if brain alterations are progressive, it is suggestive of an ongoing pathological process possibly amenable to treatment. Some studies have observed a relationship between prolonged duration of untreated psychosis and gray matter loss. First-episode patients also have less prominent structural brain abnormalities than chronically ill patients. Prospective follow-up studies of first-episode patients suggest continued gray matter loss during the first few years of the illness. Based on such findings, it has been argued that psychosis may be 'toxic' to the brain. If true, early intervention with antipsychotic drugs (APDs) could halt the progression of brain abnormalities in schizophrenia and related psychoses, and translate into favorable clinical outcome.

Since the first episode of schizophrenia is frequently preceded by subtle psychotic-like symptoms and social withdrawal (the prodromal phase), one wonders whether the structural brain changes may emerge in parallel to the functional decline that characterizes this period. Individuals at high genetic risk for developing psychosis have structural alterations such as amygdala–hippocampal and thalamic volume reductions. Prospective studies have shown that high-risk individuals who later became psychotic have less gray matter in a variety of brain regions (right medial temporal, lateral temporal, inferior frontal cortex, and cingulate cortex bilaterally). This is very suggestive of an active disease process taking place during the transition to psychosis.

Neurochemical alterations

The conventional teaching over the past decades has been that psychotic symptoms are related to excess of dopamine. Supporting this view is the fact that all effective antipsychotics block dopamine (Figure 20.3), and the fact that agents which increase dopamine levels, such as amphetamine and cocaine, can cause psychotic symptoms. Direct evidence for the dopamine hypothesis, however, has been lacking. There is indirect support based on observations of increased levels of homovanillic acid, a dopamine metabolite, in the cerebrospinal fluid of schizophrenic patients. Postmortem studies of dopamine receptor density have yielded inconsistent results. Recent positron emission tomography (PET) studies, however, support pre- and postsynaptic alterations of dopamine transmission in schizophrenia.

A more refined theory of dopamine abnormality has been proposed by Daniel Weinberger of the National Institute of Medical Health (USA), in which it is proposed that negative and cognitive symptoms in schizophrenia

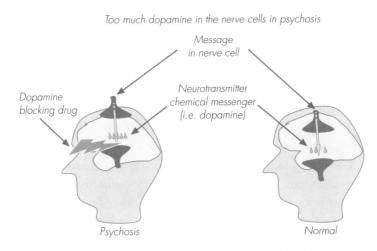

Too much dopamine in the nerve cells in psychosis

Message in nerve cell

Dopamine blocking drug

Neurotransmitter chemical messenger (i.e. dopamine)

Psychosis

Normal

Figure 20.3 The classical **dopamine excess theory** of schizophrenia. It is generally believed that psychosis is related to an excess of neurotransmitter release by the dopaminergic neurons (left) by comparison with healthy persons (right). This view is consistent with the observation that all antipsychotic drugs have an effect of blocking one or other type of dopamine receptor to a greater or lesser extent.

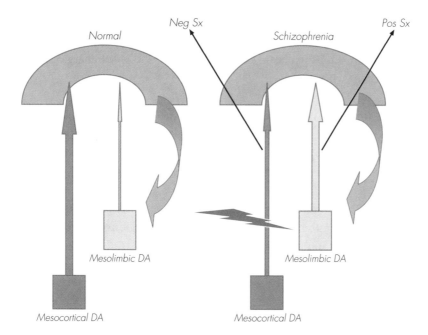

Figure 20.4 Revised dopamine hypothesis of schizophrenia (after Weinberger 1987).

may be related to hypodopaminergic activity in the mesocortical dopamine system, and that the positive symptoms may be related to a hyperdopaminergic state in the mesolimbic dopamine system (Figure 20.4). The mesolimbic system is normally inhibited by the mesocortical dopamine system; thus, the mesolimbic over-activity may be due to disinhibition from the cortical 'brakes'.

A variety of neurotransmitters are likely involved in the pathogenesis of schizophrenia. It is also possible that more fundamental defects, perhaps in cellular membranes, may be implicated. For each of these alternative hypotheses, varying degrees of evidence are available.

Serotonin. Other neurotransmitter systems have been implicated as well. The potential role of serotonin (5-hydroxytryptamine, 5-HT) in schizophrenia was discovered when lysergic acid diethylamide (LSD) resulted in psychosis. Drugs such as clozapine that block 5-HT as well as dopamine are highly effective for schizophrenia.

Noradrenaline (norepinephrine). Several investigators have implicated an increased activity of the noradrenergic system in schizophrenia. Observations that some antipsychotic drugs block α_1 and α_2 – adrenergic receptors are consistent with this view.

Gamma-amino butyric acid (GABA). Loss of GABA, an inhibitory neurotransmitter, interneurons has been observed in the hippocampus and the cingulate in schizophrenia. Such impairment in GABA inhibitory inputs could lead to an over-activity of the dopaminergic systems.

Glutamate. Glutamate, an excitatory neurotransmitter, is the most abundant neurotransmitter. Phencyclidine, a glutamatergic receptor antagonist, causes symptoms similar to schizophrenia.

Cell membrane alterations. It has been proposed that alterations in neuronal membrane structure and function may occur in schizophrenia, and that such abnormalities may explain the receptor and neurotransmitter dysregulation in this illness. Evidence has been mostly from studies of peripheral cells such as erythrocytes, although recent *in vivo* phosphorus spectroscopy studies have provided some evidence of membrane alterations in the brain.

Neurophysiological alterations

Patients with schizophrenia have a variety of alterations suggestive of dysfunction of a widely distributed network of brain regions mediating higher cognitive functions reflected in:

- reduced activation of the prefrontal cortex while performing cognitive tasks detected by PET and single photon emission tomography (SPECT) scans, as well as functional MRI;
- abnormalities in smooth pursuit eye movement (SPEM) functioning, which reflects impaired integrity of prefrontal structures that subserve eye movements;
- decreased amounts of delta sleep;
- decreased amplitude of the P300 event-related potentials;
- decreased habituation of the P50 evoked response.

Neuropathological evidence

While 19th century studies failed to find any abnormalities in postmortem brains of schizophrenia patients, recent studies have revealed the following:

- subtle reductions in cerebral volume and thinning of the cerebral cortex
- selective reductions in the volume of the thalamus
- reductions in medial temporal cortical volume.

Histopathological studies have revealed:

- reduced neuronal size
- reduced dendritic density
- decreased concentrations of synaptic proteins such as synaptophysins
- possible increased neuronal packing density
- gliosis is characteristically absent in schizophrenia.

These findings have suggested the possibility that in schizophrenia there are reductions in synaptic neuropil, perhaps related to the processes of exaggerated synaptic pruning that happens normally during adolescence.

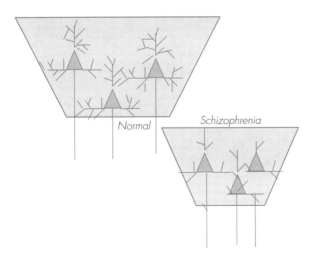

Figure 20.5 Neuronal density and decreased synapse density in schizophrenia.

When might the illness really begin?

Clarifying when schizophrenia begins (and 'what') will be essential to instituting appropriate early interventions to either mitigate its severity or even prevent its clinical emergence. Which neurodevelopmental model best explains the progression of the disorder is a vital question.

One view, the so-called early (or 'doomed from the womb') developmental model suggests that abnormalities in brain development around or before birth mediate the failure of brain functions in early adulthood. This model is supported by an array of data, such as an increased rate of birth complications, minor physical abnormalities, neurological soft signs, and subtle behavioral abnormalities in children who later developed schizophrenia. However, only a small number of people with such risk indicators eventually develop schizophrenia.

An alternative view, suggested by the fact that the illness onset does not begin typically until adolescence or early adulthood, points to a possible developmental problem around or prior to the onset of psychosis. Normally, adolescence is characterized by a refinement of neuronal connections leading to an elimination (or 'pruning') of surplus synapses. If this process is excessive, then a pronounced loss of synapses, perhaps of the glutamatergic system, may result, leading to the emergence of the illness.

Finally, the observation that at least a subgroup of patients deteriorate

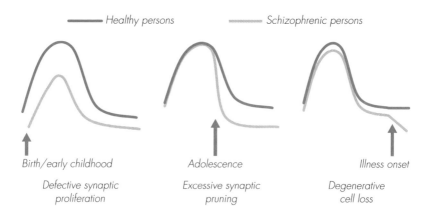

Figure 20.6 Developmental and degenerative models of schizophrenia.

over the first few years of the illness has led to the view that there may be a degenerative process.

These pathophysiological models (Figure 20.6) are not necessarily mutually exclusive. A sequential combination of these processes is possible. Environmental factors such as illicit drug use and psychosocial stress may also be potential secondary triggers accompanying the onset and course of schizophrenia.

chapter 21

What does the future hold?

Prediction is very difficult, especially of the future. Neils Bohr (1885–1962)

As for the future, your task is not to foresee it, but to enable it.
Antoine de Saint-Exupery (1900–1944)

Our task in the present is to do the best we can for our patients and their families. The future, judging from the recent past, looks hopeful. It is important to maintain an optimistic outlook, for there is good cause. There continue to be advancements on many fronts – molecular genetics, integrative biology, refined psychosocial interventions, functional brain imaging, services research, complementary medicine, prevention studies, and cross-national studies, to name but a few areas. These advancements will eventually translate into more effective and safer treatments.

Drug development

The history of pharmacological treatments has largely been one of serendipity. The future of psychopharmacology, however, is likely to be one of 'designer' drugs. It is now possible to screen thousands of molecules to identify a handful that have the possibility of becoming viable treatments. Regardless of whether a drug is devised or discovered, there are mechanisms by which safety, tolerability, and efficacy have to be established prior to releasing it for general use. In the USA, the Federal Drug Administration (FDA) serves this purpose.

All drugs go through a set of rigorously conducted studies. The first stage is preclinical studies in the laboratory to comprehensively assess safety and biological activity of the test drug; this process can take 3–4 years. The next stage is a series of clinical trials (phases) which can last 6 years or more.

Phase I trials are conducted in small groups of people (20–80) to assess safety, dosage range, and possible side effects.

Phase II trials are larger studies (100–300 individuals) to assess efficacy and safety.

Phase III trials are large-scale studies (1000–3000 individuals), frequently multi-country, to confirm efficacy, compare with placebo or standard treatments, and monitor safety.

After the completion of the trials the data is submitted to the FDA. After much deliberation about the drug's safety, efficacy, risk–benefit ratio, manufacturing methods, etc., the FDA may decide to approve the drug or request additional data. Once approved, which may take up to 12 years from the initial chemical identification, the drug is marketed. There are **phase IV** trials for some drugs to continue evaluating effectiveness and safety. The success rate of getting a potential drug off a laboratory shelf into a patient's hands is quite low. It is estimated that for every 5000 compounds screened, 5 make it to clinical trials, and 1 gets approved (1 : 5000 = 0.02% chance of success)!

There are a number of promising compounds in the pipeline, some taking the well-trodden path of 5-hydroxytryptamine (5-HT)/dopamine (DA) antagonism while others have novel mechanisms of action. Table 21.1 is a partial listing of some compounds at various stages of testing.

Prevention of schizophrenia

This is an exciting and intense area of research. Advances in understanding the developmental aspects of the disorder are now beginning to provide the impetus for prevention as a plausible goal.

It is increasingly evident that the 'seeds' of schizophrenia are planted early in the neurodevelopmental process eventually leading to deviant brain functioning, resulting in schizophrenia in late adolescence or early adulthood. It is also evident that *multiple* and *sequential* etiological factors may interactively and additively contribute to the emergence of the illness. This view

Table 21.1 Some drugs in development

Compound	Mechanism of action
Asenapine	5-HT/D_2 antagonist
Bifeprunox	Partial DA agonist/antagonist; 5-HT agonist
CX-516	AMPAkine
D-Serine	Stimulates NMDA receptors
Galantamine	Enhances cholinergic function
Glycine	Stimulates NMDA receptors
Iloperidone	DA, 5-HT, and norepinephrine antagonist
Lamotrigine	Sodium channel blocker
Memantine	NMDA receptor antagonist
Modafinil	Increases dopamine levels in the pre-frontal cortex
Ocaperidone	DA/5HT antagonist
Paliperidone	Active metabolite of risperidone
RG1068	Synthetic human secretin compound
Seromycin/d-cycloserine	Partial NMDA receptor agonist
Talnetant	Neurokinin-3 antagonist
Tolcapone	*COMT* gene inhibitor in the medial prefrontal cortex

NMDA = N-methyl-D-aspartate; AMPA = α-amino-3-hydroxy-5-methyl-4-isoxazole propionic acid

suggests that preventive treatments can be tailored to the stage of evolution of the disease process. Thus, a critical task towards this end is the identification of risk factors that assist in accurate selection of at-risk individuals for application of preventative strategies.

Primary prevention
Preventing the emergence of the disorder in at-risk persons is what the future is going to be about; currently it is a theoretical concept. It may eventually be possible to design specific interventions for genetically at-risk individuals who display biobehavioral precursors that are predictive of later illness.

Secondary prevention
Preventing full-blown psychosis in individuals at the very early phases of the illness is moving closer to reality. It is now possible to apply operational criteria to diagnose the prodromal state. The view that the subtle, psychotic-like symptoms that characterize the prodromal phase might be mediated by spurts of dopaminergic excess has encouraged early treatment with low

doses of DA-blocking drugs. In a single-blind design, McGorry and colleagues (2002) compared low-dose risperidone plus cognitive behavior therapy with a needs-based intervention (i.e. counseling and case management) for 6 months. The combined specific intervention led to a significant preventive treatment effect in 59 participants. Using a double-blind, multisite approach, Woods and colleagues (2003) compared the efficacy of olanzapine plus supportive and family therapy versus supportive and family therapy alone for one year of active treatment. Short-term data (8 weeks) suggested an improvement in symptoms associated with olanzapine treatment, although significant weight gain was also seen. There are several ongoing studies that ought to shed light on the value of secondary prevention.

Preventive approaches, particularly those utilizing antipsychotic drugs (APDs), are fraught with ethical dilemmas. For example, using APDs, even at low dose, in persons who exhibit risk behaviors but may never have gone on to develop schizophrenia is a particularly troublesome issue. It is likely that non-APD treatments may need to be developed hand-in-hand with better prediction capability.

What is needed, of course, is more research to provide definite evidence in order to rest the many hypotheses and speculations that abound.

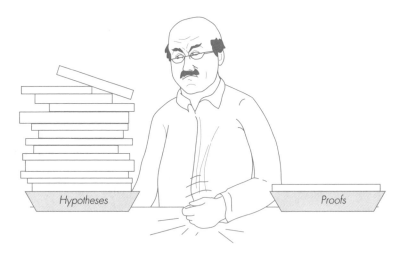

Figure 21.1 Enough theories, more proofs!

Glossary of terms

When there are several meanings of words, as is often the case, we have chosen the ones that are relevant to the topic at hand, namely schizophrenia.

Acting-out	Expressing emotional conflict or stress through behavior and actions without reflection or regard for (usually negative) consequences.
Affect	Observable behavior that reflects the experienced emotion.
Affective blunting	AKA blunted affect. Significant reduction in affective expression.
Agranulocytosis	Granulocyte count below 500/mm^3.
Akathisia	Subjective feeling of motor restlessness (jitteriness) felt mostly in the legs, often accompanied by inability to sit still or lie quietly.
Allele	One or more alternative forms of the same gene occupying a given position (locus) on a chromosome. Each person inherits two alleles for each gene, one from each parent.
Alogia	Speech that is characterized by brief and simple responses and little spontaneous speech; also called 'poverty of speech'.
Anorgasmia	Inability to achieve orgasm, even with adequate stimulation.
Association (genetics)	The relationship between specific alleles and illness in unrelated individuals (contrast with linkage). If the

frequency of the specific allele in the disease population is greater than in the unrelated control population, the allele is *in association* with the disease.

Athetosis
Recurrent stream of slow, writhing movements, typically of the hands and feet; one of the movement types seen in tardive dyskinesia.

Attention
A cognitive process of selectively concentrating on one thing in a sustained manner while ignoring other stimuli. Impaired attention leads to distractibility.

Autistic thinking
Morbid self-absorption with fantastic thinking without regard to reality; one of Bleuler's 'Four As'.

Body mass index (BMI)
A measure of body fat (weight in kilograms divided by square of height in meters). BMI between 25 and 30 is defined as overweight, 30 or more is considered obese.

Brain regions

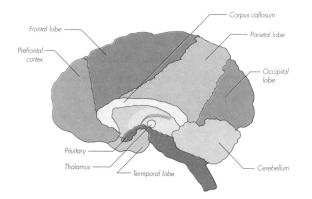

Capgras syndrome
Characterized by the belief that persons or animals of emotional significance or themselves in a mirror are impostors. Rarely, this belief extends to inanimate objects. Named after the French psychiatrist, Jean Marie Joseph Capgras (1873–1950).

Catatonia
Greek *katatonos*, stretching tight. Motor abnormalities that include catatonic stupor (a general absence of motor activity) and catatonic excitement (violent, hyperactive behavior directed at oneself or others, but with no visible purpose).

Chorea
Greek *khoreia*, choral dance. Involuntary irregular, abrupt, rapid movements involving limbs, face, and

trunk, that can result in lurching gait (hence, 'dance-like').

Circumstantiality
Speech pattern characterized by understandable, but digressive speech with irrelevant details that delays, but does not prevent, reaching its goal.

Closed-ended question
Closed-ended questions limit responses to a pre-existing set of dichotomous answers (*Did you watch TV last night?*) or can be answered in a few words. These questions can be presuming, probing, or leading.

Cognition
Latin *cognitus*, to learn, from *gno*, Indo-European roots; a broad term referring to mental processes of knowing, including aspects such as awareness, perception, reasoning, and judgment.

Cotard's delusion
Characterized by the nihilistic delusion that the person is dead or does not exist. Named after Jules Cotard (1840–1889), a French neurologist.

CT
Computed tomography (CT) or computerized axial tomography (CAT) creates an image by using an array of individual X-ray sensors that spin around the patient, permitting data from multiple angles. A computer processes this information to create an image.

Culture
The totality of socially transmitted behavior patterns, arts, beliefs, institutions, and all other products of human work and thought.

Cytochrome P450
A family of enzymes, primarily in the liver, responsible for phase I (oxidative) metabolism of drugs. Of the 40–50 isozymes, A2, 2C9, 2C19, 2D6, 3A3, 3A4 are responsible for the metabolism of a majority of psychotropic drugs, particularly 2D6 and 3A4.

Declarative memory
It is the component of memory that stores facts and events. This type of information is easily forgotten and requires repetition to long-term retention.

Decompensation
Clinical worsening from current level of stability that does not meet criteria for relapse, is transitory and fluid. The clinical worsening can spontaneously return to previous level of stability without active intervention or progress to a relapsed state.

Delirium

A reversible altered state of consciousness, characterized by confusion, disorientation, disordered thinking and memory, defective perception, prominent hyperactivity, agitation, and autonomic nervous system alterations. The DSM has specific diagnostic criteria.

Delusion

A fixed, false belief that is held in spite of evidence to the contrary, is at odds with the community's cultural and religious beliefs, is inconsistent with the level of education of the patient, and can be patently absurd.

Dementia

Latin *demens,* senseless; dementia is characterized by loss of memory, confusion, problems with understanding, and often associated with changes in personality and behavior. The DSM has specific diagnostic criteria.

Dendrites

Greek and Indo-European roots, *deru,* tree; short, highly branched fibers that carry signals *toward* the cell body of a neuron.

Denial

Defense mechanism by which unpleasant internal or external realities are kept out of conscious awareness, thus avoiding anxiety.

Derailment

AKA loosening of associations. It is a pattern of speech characterized by ideas moving from one to another in an unrelated manner. The shifts in topics are idiosyncratic.

Dermatoglyphics

The study of the skin ridges on fingertips and palms of the hands, and soles of the feet. These have been used as 'archeological' evidence of developmental events *in utero* in the case of developmental disorders, including schizophrenia.

Disease

A condition in which the functioning of the body or a part of the body is interfered with or damaged. In a person with an infectious disease, the infectious agent that has entered the body causes it to function abnormally in some way or ways. The type of abnormal functioning that occurs is the disease. Usually, the body will show some signs and symptoms of the problems it is having with functioning. Disease should not be confused with infection (from Centers of Disease Control).

Disorder	Any deviation from the normal structure or function of any part, organ, or system of the body that is manifested by a characteristic set of symptoms and signs whose pathology and prognosis may be known or unknown (from Centers of Disease Control).
Dominant	An allele that dominates or masks another allele when two different forms are present. Dominant alleles are represented by capital letters (e.g. <u>A</u>a).
Double-bind theory	An outdated theory by Gregory Bateson (1956) about the origin of schizophrenia symptoms; they are thought to be the expression of social interactions characterized by repeated exposure to conflicting messages (usually, affection on the verbal level and animosity on the nonverbal level), without the opportunity to 'escape' from them.

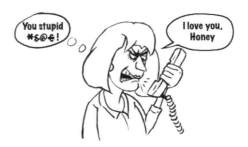

Double-blind trial	A type of (clinical) trial in which neither the volunteer nor the investigator knows what treatment the volunteer is receiving, in order to minimize bias.
Downward drift hypothesis	A theory that attempts to provide a sociocultural basis for schizophrenia. This theory basically states that, given the level of functional impairment that occurs and is necessary for diagnosis, this impairment will also occur in functional and occupational areas of life and lead to a downward drift in socioeconomic status.
Dyskinesia	Abnormal involuntary movements, including athetosis and chorea.
Dysphoria	A feeling of unpleasantness, unease, and emotional discomfort.
Dystonia	Acute muscular spasms, particularly of the tongue,

	jaw, eyes, and neck, and sometimes of the whole body.
Echolalia	Greek *lalia*, speech. Senseless repetition (echoing) of words or phrases of others, immediately after their utterance or later.
Echopraxia	Greek *praxis*, action. Senseless imitating or mirroring (echoing) the movements of others.
Effectiveness	The measure of a desired result from an intervention under usual clinical conditions. In other words: does the treatment work when used under ordinary circumstances?
Efficacy	The measure of a specific desired effect resulting from an intervention, usually under ideal experimental conditions (not the same as effectiveness).
Emotion	Latin *movere*, to move. Expression of spontaneously arising internal states of being, often associated by physiological changes. Basic emotions include anger, disgust, fear, joy, sadness, surprise. However, there is little consensus regarding what constitute basic emotions.
Empathy	Appreciation of another's problems and feelings without experiencing the same emotional reaction.
Empirical	Greek *empeirikos*, experienced. Based upon observation or experience, and capable of being tested by observation or experiment.
Endophenotype	AKA intermediate phenotype. A *heritable* trait or characteristic that is not a direct symptom of the condition but is associated with that condition.
Epidemiologic Catchment Area (ECA) study	Epidemiologic Catchment Area (ECA) was a longitudinal study, from 1980–85, which collected data on the prevalence and incidence of mental disorders in New Haven, Baltimore, St Louis, Durham and Los Angeles. A total of 20 861 patients were studied. The study provided the first definitive look at the state of mental health in the USA.
Erotomania	A delusional belief that another person, usually of a higher social status, is in love with them.
Ethnicity	The classification of a population that shares a common culture and national origin.

Executive functions	Higher order cognitive functions involved in setting goals, planning, self-regulating, and completing an intended task.
Expressed emotion	Negative communication by family members involving excessive criticism, emotional over-involvement, and intrusiveness directed at a patient.
Extrapyramidal	Related to controlling and coordinating movement by the basal ganglia.
Faith	The relational aspects of religion. Among its many meanings are: loyalty to a religion or religious community or its tenets, commitment to a relationship with God, and belief in the existence of God.
Flat affect	Absent or almost absent affective expression.
Flight of ideas	Speech characterized by abrupt changes from topic to topic, generally with comprehensible associations.
fMRI	Functional MRI used to measure hemodynamic signals related to neural activity, by taking advantage of changes in the blood flow (and oxygenation) in such areas.
Gender	Perception of masculine or feminine, which is largely culturally determined, in contrast to the biological sex.
Gliosis	Proliferation of glia in damaged areas of the central nervous system ('scarring').
Grandiosity	Inflated self-estimation (worth, power, importance, knowledge, position) which can reach delusional proportions.
Graphesthesia	The ability to recognize writing on the palm of the hand or fingertips while eyes closed; disturbance in this ability (*agraphesthesia*) may indicate deficits in the contralateral sensory cortex.
Gustatory	Latin *gustatio*, taste; pertaining to sense of taste.
Hallucination	False sensory perception in the absence of an external stimulus.
Heritability	Proportion of the observed variation in a particular phenotype-attributable to the genotype.
Hyperprolactinemia	Increased levels of prolactin in the blood (normal: less than 20 ng/ml for women, and less than 15 ng/ml for men).

Hypochondria   False belief that one is suffering from a serious illness.

Hypofrontality   Reduction in prefrontal activity, measured by regional cerebral blood flow (rCBF) or PET; hypofrontality has been observed in schizophrenia.

Ideas of reference   Incorrect interpretations of innocuous incidents or belief that external events are of personal significance.

Illusion   Distortion of sensory perception in the presence of an external stimulus.

Incidence   Number of newly diagnosed cases during a specific time period.

Insight   Awareness and understanding of the origin and meaning of one's attitudes, feelings, and behaviors and their effect on the person's environment (people and situations).

Labile, lability   Abnormal variability in affect with abrupt and unpredictable shifts.

Leukopenia   Decrease in total number of leukocytes (down to $4000-5000/mm^3$).

Lifetime prevalence   The number of individuals in the population who will develop the disorder at some point during their lifetime.

Linkage   Tendency for alleles at different loci to be inherited together. Thus, two 'linked' alleles will more likely be inherited together. This observation is taken advantage of in linkage studies in which co-segregation of the disease and genetic marker within families is examined.

Lobotomy   Outmoded surgical interruption of nerve tracts to and from the frontal lobe with the aim of treating intractable disorders such as schizophrenia and depression. The method was introduced by the Portuguese neurologist Egas Moniz in 1936, for which he was awarded the Nobel Prize.

Loose associations   Thinking characterized by tenuous connection between one thought (usually a sentence) and the next. When severe, speech becomes completely incomprehensible.

Magical thinking   Belief that one's thoughts, words, or actions can result in outcome that defies normal laws of cause and effect.

Mannerisms	Goal-directed behaviors carried out in an odd or stilted fashion.
Morbid risk	The likelihood that an individual will develop a disease during a specific period or between specific ages.
MRI	Magnetic resonance imaging; see also fMRI.
Multifactorial	When a phenotype determined by multiple genetic *and* non-genetic factors.
Myth	Greek *mythos*, a secret word or speech. Story or body of stories based on tradition or legend about the origins of the world, the causes of natural events, and the origins of the society's customs and practices.
Negative symptoms	A cluster of symptoms characterized by diminution of mental function, frequently accompanied by motor symptoms (alogia, affective flattening, anhedonia, asociality, avolition and apathy, and attentional impairment).
Neologism	Invention of word or the highly idiosyncratic use of a standard word ('my skull was completely fenestrated').
Neuroleptic	A compound that has both antipsychotic and extrapyramidal effects. The term was coined in 1952 by J. Delay who introduced chlorpromazine to psychiatry.
Neuropil	Brain tissue that lies between the neurons.
Neutropenia	Decreased neutrophils in the peripheral blood. The absolute neutrophil count (ANC) defines neutropenia, derived by multiplying the percentage of bands and neutrophils on a differential by the total white blood cell count. An abnormal ANC is fewer than 1500 cells per mm^3.
Nosology	Greek *nosos*, disease. The classification of diseases.
Olfaction	The sense of smell.
Open-ended question	A question that allows free-flowing responses (i.e. in their own words).
Orthostatic hypotension	Drop in systolic and diastolic pressures leading to postural symptoms (lightheadedness).

Overvalued idea	An unreasonable belief that is held with less than delusional intensity, and is at odds with the community's cultural and religious beliefs.
P50	Brain electrical responses to discrete stimuli can be measured by EEG, called event-related potentials (ERP). The ERP waveform contains several components including the latency period after a stimulus. Thus, P50 is an early component of the ERP, '50' representing 50 ms after the stimulus. P200 and P300 represent longer periods. These measurements have been used in schizophrenia research to study cognitive processes.
Paranoia	Irrational fear, suspicion, or distrust of others that may reach delusional proportions.
Paraphrenia	In general, refers to late-onset schizophrenia (after the age of 45 years).
Parkinsonism	Having the characteristics of Parkinson's disease (resting tremor, rigidity, bradykinesia, postural instability, and shuffling gait).
Penetrance	The extent to which the properties controlled by a gene are expressed. *Incomplete penetrance* is when less than 100% of the gene's properties are expressed in an individual.
Perception	The process of acquiring, interpreting, and organizing sensory information from the environment or one's own body.
Perinatal	The period that includes fetal and neonatal periods, defined currently as from 20 weeks' gestation to 28 days after birth.
Perseveration	The persistence of verbal or motor response from a *previous* task occurring in the current task.
PET	Positron emission tomography (PET) is a method for imaging cerebral blood flow (presumed to reflect brain activity) by using radioactive tracers that emit positrons, which are injected into the bloodstream.
Phenomenology	Refers to the study of clinical phenomena, primarily signs and symptoms.
Point prevalence	The number of individuals in a population affected by a particular disease at a single point in time.

Polygenic	Phenotype caused by the interaction of multiple genes, each of which has a relatively small effect.
Polymorphism	Variation in the structure of the gene (DNA sequences) among 1–2% of the population, permitting genetic linkage analyses.
Positive symptoms	The productive symptoms seen in schizophrenia (delusions, hallucinations, thought disorder).
Posturing	The assumption of odd postures.
Poverty of <u>content</u> of speech	Speech is adequate or even excessive in amount, but conveys little information because it is overinclusive, vague, concrete, and repetitive.
Poverty of speech	Speech is characterized by brief and simple responses and little spontaneous speech; also called alogia.
Premorbid	Preceding the onset of illness.
Prevalence	Frequency of new and old (live) cases within a population at a given time point.
Primitive reflexes	AKA infantile responses. These are a group of reflex (motor) responses found during early development; most of these reflexes are inhibited during maturation, but can be 'released' in adulthood by cerebral damage. Examples of infantile responses that later inhibited: sucking, startle, grasp, step and crawl.
Prognosis	Greek, *pro+gnosis*, foretelling. Predicting the probable course of disease.
Proprioception	Latin *proprius*, one's own. Awareness of the position of parts of the body in space in relation to one another.
Pruning	More properly *synaptic pruning*, which is normal elimination of synapses in the brain. The synapses and neurons most activated during growth are preserved.
Psychoeducation	Education (for patient and family) that serves the goals of treatment and rehabilitation; it includes information about the illness and its treatment, identifying signs of relapse, coping strategies, and problem-solving skills.
Psychosis	Psychosis is a state characterized by loss of contact with reality, with a variety of manifestations – false beliefs (delusions), false perceptions (hallucinations), irrational thinking and behaviors.

Q–Tc interval	Q–T interval represents the duration of ventricular depolarization and subsequent repolarization. Q–T interval prolongation is associated with cardiac arrhythmias. Because the Q–T interval varies with heart rate, the Q–T interval is 'normalized' into a heart-rate independent 'corrected' value, the Q–Tc interval.
Race	Distinct human populations commonly distinguished on the basis of skin color, facial features, ancestry, genetics, or national origin.
Recessive	Gene or trait that does not express in the presence of a dominant gene; two copies of the recessive gene are required for expression; indicated by lower-case letters (e.g. A<u>a</u>).
Recovery	The absence of symptoms and return to premorbid level of functioning. Some definitions also include no further requirement for treatment and no longer being viewed as psychiatrically ill.
Relapse	It is generally understood to mean clinical worsening that requires active intervention, ranging from adjustment of APD dose to hospitalization.
Relativism	A view that humans understand and evaluate beliefs and behaviors in terms of a cultural context.
Religion	The belief in the supernatural, sacred, or divine, and the moral codes, practices, values, and institutions associated with such belief. Or we might say that religion is a belief in spiritual beings; but most understand religion to mean organized religion, for example Buddhism, Christianity, Hinduism, Islam, and Judaism.
Restricted affect	Observable reduction in affective expression, not as severe as blunted affect.
Self-efficacy	The ability to cope with a situation; a concept that is important in the self-management of schizophrenia.
Sex	Male or female, identified on the basis of genetic and physical or biological characteristics.
Sialorrhea	Drooling or excessive salivation; the pooling of saliva beyond the margin of the lip.

Single-blind design	A type of (clinical) trial in which the subject does not know what treatment he or she is receiving, in order to minimize expectation.
Smooth pursuit eye movements (SPEM)	Slow eye movements that function to maintain a slowly moving image on the fovea by matching eye velocity to target velocity.
Soft signs	Neurological soft signs are minor ('soft') neurological abnormalities in sensory and motor performance identified by clinical examination. 'Soft', as opposed to 'hard', reflects the absence of any obvious localized underlying neurological pathology.
Somatic	Perception of a physical experience localized within the body.
Somatosensory	Perception originating elsewhere in the body other than in the special sense organs (e.g. eyes).
SPECT	Single photon emission computed tomography (SPECT) is a method of brain scanning using radioactive dyes (that emit gamma rays), showing areas of increased metabolic activity. It is less specific than PET.
Spirituality	Often used interchangeably with religion, may or may not include belief in supernatural beings and powers, as in religion, but emphasizes experience at a personal level, as in faith. Spirituality can mean a feeling of connectedness, feeling that life has purpose and that personal development can occur with these perspectives.
Stereognosis	The ability to recognize an object placed in the palm of the hand while eyes closed; disturbance in this ability (*asterognosis*) may indicate deficits in the contralateral sensory cortex.
Stereotypies	Non-purposeful and uniformly repetitive motions, such as tapping or rocking.
Stigma	Greek *stigma*, mark. A mark of disgrace; sign of moral blemish; stain or reproach.
Syndrome	Group or recognizable pattern of signs and symptoms or phenomena that indicate a particular trait or disease; the presence of one feature of the group alerts to the presence of the others.

Tangentiality | Thought disturbance in which thoughts/speech start off linearly, but quickly digress to unrelated areas without returning to the original point.

Tardive dyskinesia (TD) | Late (tardive) onset abnormal movements characterized by non-rhythmic choreiform (jerky) or athetoid (slow writhing) movements typically affecting the tongue, lips, jaw, fingers, toes, and trunk. TD can be transient or permanent.

Therapeutic alliance | Collaborative relationship between patient and therapist.

Thought blocking | In mid-sentence the patient appears to have lost the train of thought.

Thought broadcasting | A sense that others can read one's thoughts.

Thought insertion | Belief or experience that outside forces or entities place thoughts into one's mind.

Titration | Stepwise increase or decrease in the dose of a medication.

Verbigeration | Frequent repetition of same word or phrase.

Volition | Commonly understood to mean the *will* towards action or choice, or motivation. Lack of motivation (*avolition*) is seen in schizophrenia, classified as one of the negative symptoms.

Word salad | Speech is characterized by unconnected words or short meaningless phrases.

Working memory | A type of memory *system* that involves the short-term retention and manipulation of information, and integration of this transformed information into existing information (not to be confused with *short-term memory* which is a component of working memory).

Medications used in treating schizophrenia

Caveat (Latin *let him beware*): In a book such as this it is impossible to be thorough enough about drug dosages, side effects and interactions. Thus, use the tables below only as guides. When preparing to use these drugs, use more comprehensive sources of information.

Table B.1 Antipsychotic drugs (APDs)

	Name	Drug class	CYP450 Metabolism	Usual daily dose (mg)	Common side effects
Atypical APD	Aripiprazole	Dihydrocarbostyril	2D6, 3A4	10–30	Headache, anxiety, insomnia, nausea and vomiting, dizziness, akathisia, sedation
	Clozapine	Dibenzodiazepine	1A2, 3A4	100–600	Sedation, orthostatic hypotension, sialorrhea, anticholinergic effects, weight gain, dyslipidemias, hyperthermia, tachycardia, seizures, agranulocytosis, new-onset diabetes mellitus (DM), diabetic ketoacidosis (DKA)
	Olanzapine	Thienobenzo-diazepine	1A2	5–20	Sedation, orthostatic hypotension, weight gain, dyslipidemias, new-onset DM, dyskinesia, DKA
	Quetiapine	Dibenzothiazepine	3A4	150–900	Sedation, orthostatic hypotension, transient weight gain, dyslipidemias, new-onset DM, DKA
	Risperidone	Benzisoxazole	2D6, 3A4	2–6	Extrapyramidal side effects (EPS), increased prolactin, sedation, orthostatic hypotension, weight gain, dyslipidemias, new-onset DM, DKA
	Ziprasidone	Benzothiazolyl-piperazine	Primarily aldehyde oxidase; 3A4	40–160	Q–Tc prolongation, sedation, orthostatic hypotension, new-onset DM, DKA

Typical APDs				
Chlorpromazine	Aliphatic phenothiazine	2D6	150–1000	Sedation, orthostatic hypotension, EPS, photosensitivity, jaundice, tardive dyskinesia (TD), seizures, agranulocytosis, anticholinergic effects, weight gain
Fluphenazine	Piperazine phenothiazine	2D6	2–20	EPS, TD, weight gain
Haloperidol	Butyrophenone	3A4	2–25	EPS, TD, weight gain
Loxapine	Dibenzazepine	1A2, 2D6, 3A4	30–150	Sedation, orthostatic hypotension, EPS, TD, seizures, anticholinergic effects, weight gain
Perphenazine	Piperazine phenothiazine	2D6	16–64	Sedation, orthostatic hypotension, EPS, TD, seizures, anticholinergic effects, weight gain
Pimozide	Diphenylbutyl-piperidine	3A4	2–12	EPS, TD, weight gain
Thioridazine	Piperidine phenothiazine	2D6	100–800	Sedation, orthostatic hypotension, EPS, TD, anticholinergic effects, weight gain
Thiothixene	Thioxanthene	1A2	6–50	EPS, TD, weight gain
Trifluoperazine	Piperazine phenothiazine	2D6	5–30	Sedation, orthostatic hypotension, EPS, TD, seizures, anticholinergic effects, weight gain

Table B.2 Other drugs commonly used in treating schizophrenia

Class	Name	Common uses	Metabolism	Usual daily dose (mg)	Side effects
Antimanic	Lithium	Adjunctive; mania symptoms	Renal clearance	600–1500	Nausea & vomiting, diarrhea, tremor, weight gain, thirst, acne, polyuria, dulling, hypothyroidism, benign leukocytosis, diabetes insipidus
	Valproate	Adjunctive; mania symptoms	2C9, 2C19, other pathways	1000–1500	Nausea & vomiting, diarrhea, rash, hepatotoxicity, thrombocytopenia, pancreatitis
Antianxiety	Alprazolam	Management of acute arousal and anxiety; catatonia; management of chronic anxiety	3A3, 2C19	0.75–4	Sedation, confusion, amnesia, fatigue, blurred vision
	Clonazepam		Nitroreduction	0.5–4	
	Lorazepam		Glucuronidation	1–6	
	Buspirone	Management of chronic anxiety (non-addictive)	3A4	30–45	Headache, dizziness, gastrointestinal distress, restlessness, sedation

		Indication		Dose	Side effects
Antidepressants	Citalopram		2D6, 2C19, 3A4	20–40	Agitation, akathisia, anxiety, insomnia, gastrointestinal distress, headache, sedation, sexual dysfunction, apathy after long-term use
	Escitalopram		2D6, 2C19, 3A4	10–20	
	Fluoxetine	Depression, chronic anxiety, panic disorder, OCD	2D6, 2C9, 2C19	20–40	
	Fluvoxamine		1A2, 2D6	100–300	
	Paroxetine		2D6	20–40	
	Sertraline		3A4	50–150	
Anticholinergics	Benztropine	Parkinsonism, dystonia, akathisia, rabbit syndrome	?	2–6, 1–2 IV	Dry mouth, nose and throat, blurred vision, light sensitivity, urinary hesitancy, constipation, nausea, memory impairment, restlessness, narrow angle glaucoma, paralytic ileus, skin flushing
	Biperiden		?	4–8	
	Trihexyphenidyl		?	6–15	

Bibliography

Recommended reading

There are many classic texts that we would consider required reading. However, we think that the reader will be better served by the following review articles which provide a useful overview of the topics; most of these papers provide comprehensive bibliographies.

The books listed vary in the amount of information they include. Some were written for professionals, while others were expressly for patients and family members (we recommend that professionals read these as well so as to better understand the concerns of patients and family members).

Books

Amador X. *I am Not Sick, I Don't Need Help!* Vida Press, 2000 (ISBN: 0967718902)

American Psychiatric Association, *Practice Guidelines for the Treatment of Patients with Schizophrenia*. American Psychiatric Press, 1997

(www.psych.org/psych_pract/treatg/quick_ref_guide/SchizophreniaQRG_04–15–05.pdf)

Andreasen NC. *Brave New Brain: Conquering Mental Illness in the Era of the Genome*. Oxford University Press, 2004 (ISBN: 0195167287).

Ayd FJ. *Lexicon of Psychiatry, Neurology, and the Neurosciences,* 2nd edition. Williams & Wilkins Company 2000 (ISBN: 0781724686).

Bellack AS, Mueser KT, Gingerich S, Agresta J. *Social Skills Training for Schizophrenia: a Step-by-Step Guide*. Guilford Press, 1997 (ISBN: 157230846X).

Gottesman II. *Schizophrenia Genesis: the Origins of Madness*. WH Freeman & Co., 1990 (ISBN: 0716721473).

Harvey PD, Sharma T. *Understanding and Treating Cognition in Schizophrenia.* Martin Dunitz, 2002 (ISBN: 1841841331).

Hirsch SR, Weinberger DR, Mitchell PR (Editors). *Schizophrenia,* 2nd edition. Blackwell Publishers, 2003 (ISBN: 0632063882).

Hogarty GE. *Personal Therapy for Schizophrenia and Related Disorders: a Guide to Individualized Treatment.* Guilford Press, 2002 (ISBN: 157230782X).

Keshavan MS, Kennedy JL, Murray RM. *Neurodevelopment and Schizophrenia.* Cambridge University Press, 2004 (ISBN: 0521823315).

Lieberman JA, Murray RM. *Comprehensive Care of Schizophrenia.* Martin Dunitz, 2001 (ISBN: 1841841501).

Maxmen JS, Ward NG. *Psychotropic Drugs: Fast Facts,* 3rd edition. WW Norton & Company, 2002 (ISBN: 0393703010).

McGuffin P, Owen MJ, Gottesman II (Editors). *Psychiatric Genetics and Genomics.* Oxford University Press, 2002 (ISBN: 0192631489).

Meyer JM, Nasrallah HA. *Medical Illness and Schizophrenia.* American Psychiatric Publishing, Inc., 2003 (ISBN 1585621064).

Miller R, Mason SE. *Diagnosis: Schizophrenia.* Columbia University Press, 2002 (ISBN: 0231126255).

Othmer E, Othmer SC. *The Clinical Interview Using DSM-IV-TR. Volume 1: Fundamentals.* American Psychiatric Publishing, Inc., 2002 (ISBN 1585620513).

Othmer E, Othmer SC. *The Clinical Interview Using DSM-IV-TR. Volume 2: The Difficult Patient.* American Psychiatric Publishing, Inc., 2002 (ISBN 158562053X).

Pies RW. *Handbook of Essential Psychopharmacology,* 2nd edition. American Psychiatric Publishing, Inc., 2005 (ISBN 1585621684).

Shea S. *Psychiatric Interviewing: the Art of Understanding,* 2nd edition. WB Saunders Company, 1998 (ISBN: 0721670113).

Sheehan S. *Is There No Place on Earth for Me?* Random House, 1983 (ISBN: 0394713788).

Sims A. *Symptoms in the Mind: an Introduction to Descriptive Psychopathology.* Bailliere Tindall, 2002 (ISBN: 0702026271).

Stahl SM. *Essential Psychopharmacology: the Prescriber's Guide.* Cambridge University Press, 2004 (ISBN: 0521011698).

Torrey EF. *Surviving Schizophrenia: a Manual for Families, Consumers, and Providers,* 4th Edition. Quill, 2001 (ISBN: 0060959193).

Tseng W-S. *Clinicians Guide to Cultural Psychiatry.* Academic Press, 2003 (ISBN: 0127016333).

Articles

Arnold SE, Talbot K, Hahn CG (2005): Neurodevelopment, neuroplasticity, and new genes for schizophrenia. *Prog Brain Res* 147:319–45.

Blair IP, Mitchell PB, Schofield PR (2005): Techniques for the identification of genes involved in psychiatric disorders. *Aust NZ J Psychiatry* 39:542–9.

Braham LG, Trower P, Birchwood M (2004): Acting on command hallucinations and dangerous behavior: a critique of the major findings in the last decade. *Clin Psychol Rev* 24:513–28.

Cantor-Graae E, Selten JP (2005): Schizophrenia and migration: a meta-analysis and review. *Am J Psychiatry* 162:12–24.

Casey DE (2004): Dyslipidemia and atypical antipsychotic drugs. *J Clin Psychiatry* 65 (Suppl 18):27–35.

Fanous AH, Kendler KS (2005): Genetic heterogeneity, modifier genes, and quantitative phenotypes in psychiatric illness: searching for a framework. *Mol Psychiatry* 10:6–13.

Goff DC, Cather C, Evins AE, *et al.* (2005): Medical morbidity and mortality in schizophrenia: guidelines for psychiatrists. *J Clin Psychiatry* 66:183–94; quiz 147, 273–4.

Haddock G, Lewis S (2005): Psychological interventions in early psychosis. *Schizophr Bull* 31:697–704.

Harrison PJ, Weinberger DR (2005): Schizophrenia genes, gene expression, and neuropathology: on the matter of their convergence. *Mol Psychiatry* 10:40–68.

Hawton K, Sutton L, Haw C, Sinclair J, Deeks JJ (2005): Schizophrenia and suicide: systematic review of risk factors. *Br J Psychiatry* 187:9–20.

Holt RI, Peveler RC, Byrne CD (2004): Schizophrenia, the metabolic syndrome and diabetes. *Diabet Med* 21:515–23.

Kelly DL, Conley RR (2004): Sexuality and schizophrenia: a review. *Schizophr Bull* 30:767–79.

Kurtz MM (2005): Neurocognitive impairment across the lifespan in schizophrenia: an update. *Schizophr Res* 74:15–26.

Lee C, McGlashan TH, Woods SW (2005): Prevention of schizophrenia: can it be achieved? *CNS Drugs* 19:193–206.

McGrath J, Saha S, Welham J, El Saadi O, MacCauley C, Chant D (2004): A systematic review of the incidence of schizophrenia: the distribution of rates and the influence of sex, urbanicity, migrant status and methodology. *BMC Med* 2:13.

Miller AL, Hall CS, Buchanan RW, *et al.* (2004): The Texas Medication Algorithm Project antipsychotic algorithm for schizophrenia: 2003 update. *J Clin Psychiatry* 65:500–8.

Miyamoto S, Duncan GE, Marx CE, Lieberman JA (2005): Treatments for schizophrenia: a critical review of pharmacology and mechanisms of action of antipsychotic drugs. *Mol Psychiatry* 10:79–104.

Newcomer JW (2004): Abnormalities of glucose metabolism associated with atypical antipsychotic drugs. *J Clin Psychiatry* 65 (Suppl 18):36–46.

Northup A, Nimgaonkar VL (2004): Genetics of schizophrenia: implications for treatment. *Expert Rev Neurother* 4:725–31.

Palmer BA, Pankratz VS, Bostwick JM (2005): The lifetime risk of suicide in schizophrenia: a reexamination. *Arch Gen Psychiatry* 62:247–53.

Pantelis C, Yucel M, Wood SJ, *et al.* (2005): Structural brain imaging evidence for multiple pathological processes at different stages of brain development in schizophrenia. *Schizophr Bull* 31:672–96.

Penn DL, Mueser KT, Tarrier N, *et al.* (2004): Supportive therapy for schizophrenia: possible mechanisms and implications for adjunctive psychosocial treatments. *Schizophr Bull* 30:101–12.

Rapoport JL, Addington AM, Frangou S, Psych MR (2005): The neurodevelopmental model of schizophrenia: update 2005. *Mol Psychiatry* 10:434–49.

Robinson DG, Woerner MG, Delman HM, Kane JM (2005): Pharmacological treatments for first-episode schizophrenia. *Schizophr Bull* 31:705–22.

Sacks FM (2004): Metabolic syndrome: epidemiology and consequences. *J Clin Psychiatry* 65 (Suppl 18):3–12.

Semple DM, McIntosh AM, Lawrie SM (2005): Cannabis as a risk factor for psychosis: systematic review. *J Psychopharmacol* 19:187–94.

Tamminga CA, Holcomb HH (2005): Phenotype of schizophrenia: a review and formulation. *Mol Psychiatry* 10:27–39.

Tarrier N (2005): Cognitive behaviour therapy for schizophrenia – a review of development, evidence and implementation. *Psychother Psychosom* 74:136–44.

Taylor M, Chaudhry I, Cross M, *et al.* (2005): Towards consensus in the long-term management of relapse prevention in schizophrenia. *Hum Psychopharmacol* 20:175–81.

Wagstaff AJ, Easton J, Scott LJ (2005): Intramuscular olanzapine: a review of its use in the management of acute agitation. *CNS Drugs* 19:147–64.

Wirshing DA (2004): Schizophrenia and obesity: impact of antipsychotic medications. *J Clin Psychiatry* 65 (Suppl 18):13–26.

Selected further reading

Ananth J, Venkatesh R, Burgoyne K, Gadasalli R, Binford R, Gunatilake S (2004): Atypical antipsychotic induced weight gain: pathophysiology and management. *Ann Clin Psychiatry* 16:75–85.

Andreasen NC (1989): The Scale for the Assessment of Negative Symptoms (SANS): conceptual and theoretical foundations. *Br J Psychiatry Suppl* 7:49–58.

Andreasen NC, Carpenter WT, Jr., Kane JM, Lasser RA, Marder SR, Weinberger DR (2005): Remission in schizophrenia: proposed criteria and rationale for consensus. *Am J Psychiatry* 162:441–9.

Angermeyer MC, Matschinger H (2005): Labeling–stereotype–discrimination. An investigation of the stigma process. *Soc Psychiatry Psychiatr Epidemiol* 40:391–5.

Bertolino A, Roffman JL, Lipska BK, *et al.* (2000): Reduced N-acetylaspartate in prefrontal cortex of adult rats with neonatal hippocampal damage. *Cereb Cortex* 12(9):983–90.

Birchwood M, Smith J, Macmillan F, *et al.* (1989): Predicting relapse in schizophrenia: the development and implementation of an early signs monitoring system using patients and families as observers, a preliminary investigation. *Psychol Med* 19:649–56.

Block W, Bayer TA, Tepest R *et al.* (2000): Decreased frontal lobe ratio of N-acetyl aspartate to choline in familial schizophrenia: a proton magnetic resonance spectroscopy study. *Neurosci Lett* 289(2):147–51.

Buckley P, Miller A, Olsen J, Garver D, Miller DD, Csernansky J (2001): When symptoms persist: clozapine augmentation strategies. *Schizophr Bull* 27:615–28.

Bustillo J, Lauriello J, Horan W, Keith S (2001): The psychosocial treatment of schizophrenia: an update. *Am J Psychiatry* 158:163–75.

Cannon M, Clarke MC (2005): Risk for schizophrenia – broadening the concepts, pushing back the boundaries. *Schizophr Res* 79:5–13.

Cantwell R (2003): Substance use and schizophrenia: effects on symptoms, social functioning and service use. *Br J Psychiatry* 182:324–9.

Chovil I (2005): First psychosis prodrome: rehabilitation and recovery. *Psychiatr Rehabil J* 28:407–10.

Corrigan PW, River LP, Lundin RK, *et al.* (2001): Three strategies for changing attributions about severe mental illness. *Schizophr Bull* 27:187–95

de Leon J, Diaz FJ (2005): A meta-analysis of worldwide studies demonstrates an association between schizophrenia and tobacco smoking behaviors. *Schizophr Res* 76:135–57

Green MF (1993): Cognitive remediation in schizophrenia: is it time yet? *Am J Psychiatry* 150:178–87.

Harrison PJ, Weinberger DR (2005): Schizophrenia genes, gene expression, and neuropathology: on the matter of their convergence. *Mol Psychiatry* 10:40–68.

Heresco-Levy U, Javitt DC (2004): Comparative effects of glycine and D-cycloserine on persistent negative symptoms in schizophrenia: a retrospective analysis. Schizophr Res 66:89–96.

Hogarty GE, Flesher S (1999): Developmental theory for a cognitive enhancement therapy of schizophrenia. *Schizophr Bull* 25:677–92.

Hogarty GE, Flesher S, Ulrich R, *et al.* (2004), Cognitive enhancement therapy for schizophrenia: effects of a 2-year randomized trial on cognition and behavior. *Arch Gen Psychiatry* 61:866–76.

Keefe RS, Seidman LJ, Christensen BK *et al.* (2004): Comparative effect of atypical and conventional antipsychotic drugs on neurocognition in first-episode psychosis: a randomized, double-blind trial of olanzapine versus low doses of haloperidol. *Am J Psychiatry* 161(6):985–95.

Keshavan MS (1999): Development, disease and degeneration in schizophrenia: a unitary pathophysiological model. *J Psychiatr Res* 33:513–21.

Keshavan MS, Carter CS (2000): First-episode schizophrenia: a phase-specific approach to management. *Primary Psychiatry* 7:43–50

Keshavan MS, Schooler NR (1992): First-episode studies in schizophrenia: criteria and characterization. *Schizophr Bull* 18(3):491–513.

Keshavan MS, Anderson S, Pettegrew JW (1994): Is schizophrenia due to excessive synaptic pruning in the prefrontal cortex? The Feinberg hypothesis revisited. *J Psychiatr Res* 28(3):239–65.

Keshavan MS, Schooler NR, Sweeney JA, Haas GL, Pettegrew JW (1998): Research and treatment strategies in first-episode psychoses. The Pittsburgh experience. *Br J Psychiatry Suppl* 172:60–5.

Keshavan MS, Rabinowitz J, DeSmedt G, Harvey PD, Schooler N (2004): Correlates of insight in first episode psychosis. *Schizophr Res* 70:187–94.

Keshavan MS, Duggal HS, Veeragandham G, *et al.* (2005): Personality dimensions in first-episode psychoses. *Am J Psychiatry* 162:102–9.

Lehman AF, Lieberman JA, Dixon LB, *et al.* (2004): Practice guideline for the treatment of patients with schizophrenia, 2nd edition. *Am J Psychiatry* 161:1–56.

Leucht S, Barnes TR, Kissling W, Engel RR, Correll C, Kane JM (2003): Relapse prevention in schizophrenia with new-generation antipsychotics: a systematic review and exploratory meta-analysis of randomized, controlled trials. *Am J Psychiatry* 160:1209–22.

Lewis DA, Levitt P (2002): Schizophrenia as a disorder of neurodevelopment. *Annu Rev Neurosci* 25:409–32.

Lieberman J, Perkins D, Belger A, *et al.* (2001): The early stages of schizophrenia: speculations on pathogenesis, pathophysiology, and therapeutic approaches. [Published erratum *Biol Psychiatry* 51(4):346.] *Biol Psychiatry* 50(11):884–97.

Malla A, Payne J (2005): First-episode psychosis: psychopathology, quality of life, and functional outcome. *Schizophr Bull* 31(3):650–71.

Marder SR (2003): Overview of partial compliance. *J Clin Psychiatry* 64 (Suppl 16):3–9.

McFarlane WR, Dixon L, Lukens E, Lucksted A (2003): Family psychoeducation and schizophrenia: a review of the literature. *J Marital Fam Ther* 29:223–45.

McGorry PD, Yung AR, Phillips LJ, *et al.* (2002): Randomized controlled trial of interventions designed to reduce the risk of progression to first-episode psychosis in a clinical sample with subthreshold symptoms. *Arch Gen Psychiatry* 59(10):921–8.

Meltzer HY, Alphs L, Green AI, *et al.* (2003): Clozapine treatment for suicidality in schizophrenia: International Suicide Prevention Trial (InterSePT). *Arch Gen Psychiatry* 60:82–91.

Mohr S, Huguelet P (2004): The relationship between schizophrenia and religion and its implications for care. *Swiss Med Wkly* 134:369–76.

Murray RM, Lewis SW (1987): Is schizophrenia a neurodevelopmental disorder? *BMJ* (*Clin Res Ed*) 19(295):681–2.

Nasrallah HA, Targum SD, Tandon R, McCombs JS, Ross R (2005): Defining and measuring clinical effectiveness in the treatment of schizophrenia. *Psychiatr Serv* 56:273–82.

Newcomer JW (2004): Metabolic risk during antipsychotic treatment. *Clin Ther* 26:1936–46.

Newhouse P, Singh A, Potter A (2004): Nicotine and nicotinic receptor involvement in neuropsychiatric disorders. *Curr Top Med Chem* 4:267–82.

Ohlsen RI, O'Toole MS, Purvis RG, *et al.* (2004): Clinical effectiveness in first-episode patients. *Eur Neuropsychopharmacol* 14(4):S445-51.

Owen MJ, Williams NM, O'Donovan MC (2004): The molecular genetics of schizophrenia: new findings promise new insights. *Mol Psychiatry* 9:14–27.

Pantelis C, Lambert TJ (2003): Managing patients with "treatment-resistant" schizophrenia. *Med J Aust* 178 (Suppl):S62–6.

Pantelis C, Velakoulis D, McGorry PD, *et al.* (2003): Neuroanatomical abnormalities before and after onset of psychosis: a cross-sectional and longitudinal MRI comparison. *Lancet* 25(361):281–8

Pettegrew JW, Keshavan MS, Panchalingam K, *et al.* (1991): Alterations in brain high-energy phosphate and membrane phospholipid metabolism in first-episode, drug-naive schizophrenics. A pilot study of the dorsal prefrontal cortex by in vivo phosphorus 31 nuclear magnetic resonance spectroscopy. *Arch Gen Psychiatry* 48:563–8.

Pierre JM (2001): Faith or delusion? At the crossroads of religion and psychosis. *J Psychiatr Pract* 7:163–72.

Reddy R (2005): Simplified Clinical Assessment of Psychosis (SCAP). Version 1.1. University of Pitsburgh, PA, USA.

Saha S, Chant D, Welham J, McGrath J (2005): A systematic review of the prevalence of schizophrenia. *PLoS Med* 2:e141.

Seckinger RA, Amador XF (2001): Cognitive-behavioral therapy in schizophrenia. *J Psychiatr Pract* 7:173–84.

Seeman MV (2004): Gender differences in the prescribing of antipsychotic drugs. *Am J Psychiatry* 161:1324–33.

Sharma T, Antonova L (2003): Cognitive function in schizophrenia. Deficits, functional consequences, and future treatment. *Psychiatr Clin North Am* 26:25–40.

Thompson JL, Pogue-Geile MF, Grace AA (2004): Developmental pathology, dopamine, and stress: a model for the age of onset of schizophrenia symptoms. *Schizophr Bull* 30:875–900.

Thompson PM, Vidal C, Giedd JN, *et al.* (2001), Mapping adolescent brain change reveals dynamic wave of accelerated gray matter loss in very early-onset schizophrenia. Proc Natl Acad Sci USA 98(20):11650–5.

Turkington D, Dudley R, Warman DM, Beck AT (2004): Cognitive-behavioral therapy for schizophrenia: a review. *J Psychiatr Pract* 10:5–16.

Voruganti L, Awad AG (2004): Neuroleptic dysphoria: towards a new synthesis. *Psychopharmacology (Berl)* 171:121–32.

Walsh E, Buchanan A, Fahy T (2002): Violence and schizophrenia: examining the evidence. *Br J Psychiatry* 180:490–5.

Weinberger DR (1987): Implications of normal brain development for the pathogenesis of schizophrenia. *Arch Gen Psychiatry* 44(7):660–9.

Weinberger DR, Berman KF, Daniel DG (1992): Mesoprefrontal cortical dopaminergic activity and prefrontal hypofunction in schizophrenia. *Clin Neuropharmacol* 15 (Suppl 1, Pt A):568A-569A.

Woods SW, Breier A, Zipursky RB, *et al.* (2003): Randomized trial of olanzapine versus placebo in the symptomatic acute treatment of the schizophrenic prodrome. [Published erratum *Biol Psychiatry* 54(4):497.] *Biol Psychiatry* 54(4):453–64

Yung AR, McGorry PD, McFarlane CA, Jackson HJ, Patton GC, Rakkar A (1996): Monitoring and care of young people at incipient risk of psychosis. *Schizophr Bull* 22:283–303.

Sources of help and information

The few books listed below, in our view, are essential reading for patients and families. More extensive reading lists are provided at various schizophrenia-related websites.

Essential reading

Amador X. *I am Not Sick, I Don't Need Help!* Vida Press, 2000 (ISBN: 0967718902).

Andreasen NC. *Brave New Brain: Conquering Mental Illness in the Era of the Genome.* Oxford University Press, 2004 (ISBN: 0195167287).

Torrey, E Fuller. *Surviving Schizophrenia: a Manual for Families, Consumers, and Providers*, 4th Edition. Quill, 2001 (ISBN: 0060959193).

Websites

The Internet has been a tremendous boon to patients and practitioners alike. With increasing worldwide access to websites, people can benefit from personal experiences and research in different parts of the world at a pace that was unimaginable only a few years ago. An additional advantage of websites is the ease of updating information.

www.chovil.com
Ian Chovil shares his experience with schizophrenia, providing in the process a great deal of information and insights into the illness.

www.health.org
Contains fact sheets, research news and updates, online resource guides and a powerful search engine.

www.healthtouch.com
Find information about medications easily and quickly on this site.

www.medscape.com
This site offers daily, up-to-date information on the latest medical research.

www.mentalhealth.com
An excellent resource, this website is easy to navigate and provides information concerning disease symptoms, possible causes, diagnostic criteria and treatment.

www.mentalhealth.org
Sponsored by the US government, this site includes links to mental health and substance abuse databases and an extensive list of publications.

www.mentalwellness.com
A comprehensive site with information about schizophrenia and bipolar disorder.

www.mhsource.com
This site provides useful information on research and clinical trials in psychiatry.

www.nami.org
This is a very useful website from the National Alliance for the Mentally Ill, which is an organization of families, consumers, and professionals dedicated to the care of the mentally ill.

www.narsad.org
From the website: 'NARSAD (National Alliance for Research on Schizophrenia and Depression) is a private, not-for-profit public charity 501(C)(3) organized for the purpose of raising funds for scientific research into the causes, cures, treatments and prevention of severe psychiatric brain disorders, such as schizophrenia and depression'.

www.ncbi.nlm.nih.gov/entrez/query.fcgi?DB=pubmed
Allows search of the National Library of Medicine's database.

www.nimh.nih.gov
The National Institute of Mental Health is the largest source of support for psychiatric research.

www.prodigy.nhs.uk/guidance.asp?gt=Schizophrenia
From the website: 'This guidance is based on the National Institute for Clinical Excellence (NICE) guideline, *Schizophrenia: full national clinical guideline and core interventions in primary and secondary care*' (December 2002).

www.psych.org
The American Psychiatric Association website, which has information for professionals and the public.

www.psychguides.com
Contains the expert consensus treatment guideline for schizophrenia from 1999; guidelines for other disorders are also available.

www.psychosisresearch.org
Dr Keshavan's research website that has links to the very useful *Insight* newsletter.

www.pparx.org
Text from the site. 'The Partnership for Prescription Assistance brings together America's pharmaceutical companies, doctors, other health care providers, patient advocacy organizations and community groups to help qualifying patients who lack prescription coverage get the medicines they need through the public or private program that's right for them. Many will get them free or nearly free. Its mission is to increase awareness of patient assistance programs and boost enrollment of those who are eligible.'

www.rethink.org
A comprehensive, easy-to-navigate website about schizophrenia, located in the UK.

www.schizophrenia.com
The most comprehensive website about schizophrenia.

www.schizophreniadigest.com
From the website: 'Mr MacPhee was diagnosed with schizophrenia in 1987. After years of struggling with the devastating symptoms of the disease, the Fort Erie, Ontario resident was able to regain control of his life through medication, family support and other therapies. Recognizing the need for an informative publication, he launched *Schizophrenia Digest* magazine in March 1994.'

Schizophrenia organizations

IEPA (International Early Psychosis Association)
www.iepa.org.au

NARSAD (National Alliance for Research on Schizophrenia and Depression)
60 Cutter Mill Road, Suite 404
Great Neck, New York 11021, USA
Tel: (800) 829-8289
www.narsad.org

World Fellowship for Schizophrenia and Allied Disorders
124 Merton Street, Suite 507
Toronto, Ontario, M4S 2Z2, Canada
www.world-schizophrenia.org

Pharmaceutical companies in the USA

Patient assistance is provided by pharmaceutical companies at these telephone numbers:

Solvay Pharmaceuticals	800–256–8918
Ortho McNeil Pharmaceutical	800–577–3788
Abbot Laboratories	800–222–6885
Wyeth	800–568–9938

Merck and Co.	800–994–2111
GlaxoSmithKline	800–728–4368
AstraZeneca Pharmaceuticals	800–424–3727
Bristol-Myers Squibb Co.	800–736–0003
Novartis Pharmaceuticals Corp.	800–277–2254
Forest Pharmaceuticals	800–851–0758
Pfizer Inc.	800–707–8990
Cephalon	800–511–2120

Centers for early psychosis treatment and research

The following are a few of the centers worldwide that are known for pioneering work in early psychosis. Contact each center directly for more detailed information on research and clinical services.

NORTH AMERICA
Developmental Processes in the Early Course of Illness
Dept of Psychiatry and Biobehavioral Sciences
UCLA
405 Hilgard Ave
Los Angeles, CA 90095, USA
Tel: (310) 825-0036

EPI (Early Psychosis Intervention) Program
15521 Russell Avenue
White Rock, BC, V4B 2R4, Canada
Tel: 604-538-4278
www.psychosissucks.ca/epi

Early Psychosis Treatment and Prevention Program
Dept of Psychiatry
Foothills Hospital
1403 29 St NW
Calgary, Alberta, Canada T2N 2T9
Tel: (403) 670–4836
www.calgaryhealthregion.ca

First Episode Program
University of Illinois Hospital
912 S Wood Street
Chicago, IL 60612, USA
Tel: 312-996-7383
http://ccm.psych.uic.edu/Research/Schizophrenia/firstEpiPrgm.htm

First Episode Psychosis Program
The Clarke Institute of Psychiatry
Schizophrenia Division
250 College Street
Toronto, Ontario, Canada M5T 1R8
Tel: (416) 979–6913
www.camh.net

NSEPP (Nova Scotia Early Psychosis Program)
Dept of Psychiatry
5909 Jubilee Road
Halifax, Nova Scotia, Canada B3H 2E2
Tel: (902) 464-6501
www.cdha.nshealth.ca/programsandservices/mentalhealth/earlyPsychosis.htm

PEPP (Prevention and Early Intervention Program for Psychoses)
Dept of Psychiatry
University of Western Ontario, London
London Health Sciences Center
London, Ontario, Canada N6A 4G5
Tel: (519) 667–6773
www.pepp.ca

PRIME (Prevention through Risk Identification Management and Education)
Yale Psychiatric Institute
Yale University
184 Liberty Street
PO Box 208038
New Haven, CT 06520, USA
Tel: (203) 785–7210
http://info.med.yale.edu

RAPP (Recognition and Prevention of Psychological Problems)
Psychiatry Research
Hillside Hospital
75–59 263 Street
Glen Oaks, NY 11004, USA
Tel: (718) 470–8034
www.lij.edu/hil/rap

STEP (Services for the Treatment of Early Psychosis)
Western Psychiatric Institute and Clinic
3811 O'Hara Street
Pittsburgh, PA 15213, USA
Tel: (412) 586–9009
www.psychosisresearch.org

SOUTH AMERICA

ASAS (Avaliação e Seguimento de Adolescentes e Adultos Jovens na Cidade de São Paulo)
Rua Capote Valente, 763
Sao Paulo, Brazil
Tel: (05511) 3083-2655
www.usp.br/agen/bols/2004/rede1513.htm#tercdestaq

GIPSI (Grupo de Intervenção Precoce nas Psicoses)
University of Brasilia
SQN 216, Bloco C, Apto 511
Brasilia, Distrito Federal, Brazil

ASIA

Asian Network of Early Psychosis
http://asianep.net

Early Assessment Service for Young People with Psychosis (EASY)
Hong Kong
www.ha.org.hk

EPIP (Early Psychosis Intervention Programme)
Institute of Mental Health,
Woodbridge Hospital
10 Buangkok View
Singapore 539747
Tel: 6389 2200
www.epip.org.sg

Early Intervention Programme
Schizophrenia Research Foundation (SCARF)
R-7A North Main Road
AnnaNagar West (Extn)
Chennai 600 101
Tamil Nadu, India
Tel: +91-44-2615 3971
www.scarfindia.org

EUROPE
DELTA Project (Detection and Education and Local Team Assessment)
1 Marine Terrace
Dun Laoghaire, Dublin
Ireland
Tel: (01) 2366730

EIIP (Early Intervention in Psychosis)
Farmside (Mid), West Park, Horton Lane
Epsom, KT19 8PB, UK
Tel: 01372 206262

ETHOS (Early Intervention and Home-based Outreach Service)
Fir Tower, Springfield University Hospital,
61 Glenburnie Road, London, SW17 7DJ, UK
Tel: 020 8871 6571
www.access-it.org/ethos.html

IRIS (Initiative to Reduce the Impact of Schizophrenia)
www.iris-initiative.org.uk

LEO (Lambeth Early Onset Team)
3–6 Beale House
Lingham Street
Stockwell SW9 9HG, UK
Tel: 020 7326 2840
http://www.slam.nhs.uk/services/pages/detail.asp?id=506

OASIS (Outreach and Support in South London)
PO 67, Institute of Psychiatry
De Crespigny Park
London, UK
Tel: 020 7848 0952
www.oasislondon.com

Réseau de Soins PREPSY
Santé mentale
14-20 Rue Mathurin Régnier
75015 Paris, France
Tel: 0147837219
www.prepsy.org

SWEPP (Swiss Early Psychosis Project)
www.swepp.ch

AUSTRALIA AND NEW ZEALAND
EPPIC (Early Psychosis Prevention and Intervention Centre)
Poplar Road,
Parkville, Melbourne
Australia
Tel: 1800 888 320
www.eppic.org.au

(NEPP) Noarlunga Early Psychosis Program
Mental Health Services
Alexander Kelly Drive
Noarlunga Centre, South Australia
Tel: 08 8384 9599
www.onkaparingacity.com/services/doc-noarlunga_mental_health_services.html

Totara House Early Intervention for Psychosis Service
194 Bealey Ave
Christchurch, New Zealand
Tel: 377 9733
www.cdhb.govt.nz/totara/

Antipsychotic drug manufacturers

The following list includes primary telephone numbers (once contacted they can direct the caller to prescription assistance programs). Local telephone numbers are available at the websites.

Aripiprazole (Abilify)	Bristol-Myers Squibb Co., USA	212-546-4000	www.bms.com
Chlorpromazine (Thorazine)	GlaxoSmithKline, UK	44-020-8047-5000	www.gsk.com
Clozapine (Clozaril)	Novartis Pharmaceuticals Corp. Switzerland	41-61-324-1111	www.novartis.com
Flupenthixol (Fluanxol, Depixol)	Lundbeck, Denmark	45-36-301-311	www.lundbeck.com
Fluphenazine (Prolixin)	Apothecon, Inc. Netherlands	31-0342-426-120	www.apothecon.nl
Haloperidol (Haldol)	Ortho McNeil Pharmaceutical, USA	800-682-6532	www.ortho-mcneil.com
Loxapine (Loxitane)	Watson Pharmaceuticals	800-272-5525	www.watsonpharm.com
Olanzapine (Zyprexa, Zydis)	Eli Lilly & Co.	800-545-5979	www.lilly.com
Perphenazine (Trilafon)	Schering Corporation Germany	49-30-468-1111	www.schering.de
Pimozide (Orap)	Gate Pharmaceuticals	800-292-4283	www.gatepharma.com
Quetiapine (Seroquel)	AstraZeneca Pharmaceuticals	44-020-7304-5000	www.astrazeneca.com
Risperidone (Risperidal)	Janssen Pharmaceutica	32-3-280-5411	www.janssen.com
Thioridazine (Mellaril	Novartis Pharmaceuticals Corp Switzerland	41-61-324-1111	www.novartis.com
Thiothixene (Navane)	Pfizer Inc.	800-879-3477	www.pfizer.com
Trifluoperazine (Stelazine)	GlaxoSmithKline, UK	44-020-8047-5000	www.gsk.com
Ziprasidone (Geodon)	Pfizer Inc.	800-879-3477	www.pfizer.com
Zotepine (Zoleptil)	Orion Pharma	358-10-4291	www.orion.fi

Index